Comments and Observations by Friends

I knew Joe was working on this book. But he doesn't like to show his writing to anyone until he is done. So, it was a while before he allowed me to read it, including the part he wrote about me.

Knowing Joe and being involved in his life for the past eighteen years has been quite an experience. I had no idea way back when I met him that I would be caught-up in the three-ring circus that his life can sometimes be.

I thought disabled people lived quiet, sedate lives. Ha! I was sure wrong about that; at least as far as Joe's life was concerned. It has been one crisis, triumph, disaster, award ceremony, injury, wheelchair breakdown, care provider quitting without notice, TV interview to give, or board meeting to attend after another.

His whole existence is an absolute whirlwind of activity and people coming and going. I realize that my life is quiet and sedate, but his sure isn't.

This book gives the reader an insight into the constantly surprising, sometimes scary, and always interesting twists, turns, ups, downs, sad, and happy events in the life of an incredible guy. His days consist of just trying to arrange for his next meal, keeping up with reading books on CD, writing his stories, and not missing any of the juicy bits of life.

Linda Foster, September 22, 2010

Joe is one remarkable person. He is extremely physically handicapped from cerebral palsy. However, he has a very sharp mind. I have been one of his care providers for fourteen years. We, as care providers, make his life work. As his care provider, you have to do all of his daily care from feeding to bathing, as he cannot do these things for himself.

He has taken me to college with him to be his translator because he has a speech problem. I have learned a lot from doing this as I am sitting in his writing class with him. I am even writing a cookbook of Joe's favorite recipes and meals. It explains how to fix his food in a way that keeps the food from choking him, as he has chewing and swallowing difficulties, but also keeps the texture and favor pleasing to him.

When I am around him, we have fun. Linda, another friend and care provider, has taken the three of us on numerous trips to the mountains, including Yosemite, and over to the ocean. We have done day trips to many of the small towns here in the Central Valley and in the foothills of the Sierras. We have visited local museums, the zoo, the county fair, parks, wild life preserves, and other nearby attractions.

We have had some good times doing these things. We have come to be close friends, the three of us. However, it is getting harder to make these trips work out for us now. We are all getting older.

Joe fills your life with hope and makes you feel like trying to do anything that you want to do. He has encouraged me to improve my reading and writing abilities.

One day Joe was writing a story about a gopher. I read the story and I liked it. He wanted to give up on it. But I said don't; it will work! This book is the result.

Mable Gilstrap, September 29, 2010

iv

Keeping Up With Jerry

A collection of scenes based upon personal recollections and reflections from the life of someone who has cerebral palsy; written from the viewpoint of a gopher.

By

Joe Leroy Hemphill

Contact Information

If you wish to use any of the material contained in this book in another publication, please contact the author. It is his mission and goal to share his story, especially with young adults and the parents of young people with cerebral palsy. He is delighted to have his writings reprinted in additional publications and shared with a wider audience than he can possibly reach out to on his own.

Contact: Joe Hemphill
Email: writerjoe@sbcglobal.net

Table of Contents

Dedication

I dedicate this book to my father and mother.
They instilled in me the courage to live life to the fullest.

Cerebral Palsy: What It Is and How It Happens

Cerebral palsy is brain damage caused by lack of oxygen. In my case, this happened at birth. I didn't get enough oxygen for five minutes. This is why I have trouble walking, talking, and doing activities that require fine motor skills. Cerebral palsy can affect everyone differently. It depends upon how long they went without enough oxygen to the brain.

Other writings by Joe Leroy Hemphill

Tomorrow at Eight, a Novel

Collected Poems

Collected Short Stories

Essays and Letters to the Editor:
Cerebral Palsy Cannot Silence My Speech
Creative Mind Helps Him to Meet Daily Challenges
Backup Plans Create Havoc for Disabled
We All Need to Broaden Horizons on What's Normal
Not One Way to Communicate

xii

Introduction

When Joe was four, his mom, dad, his brother Larry, and Joe moved from Missouri to California because his dad heard that California had more opportunities for a child like Joe who had cerebral palsy. His father felt that as long as his son had the best chance at that time to grow into an independent adult, it was worth giving up the two businesses and the beautiful house he had built especially for Joe's mom in Missouri.

His folks decided early on that Joe wasn't going to use his handicap to get his own way. When he ordered his brother Larry to get a toy that Joe could have gotten on his own, Joe's dad overheard and gave him a spanking. Joe's mom, years later, told Joe that his dad went into the other room and cried after giving him that spanking. His dad passed away when Joe was twelve.

Joe and Larry's childhood was both very special and normal at the same time. Once, Larry came home from kindergarten puzzled why another boy didn't have a brother at home in a wheelchair. There was the time Larry and Joe were playing cowboys and Joe was the outlaw so Larry was going to hang him from the walnut tree in their backyard. Their mom glanced up just in time to save Joe. They both went to bed with out dinner, Larry for doing it and Joe for letting him.

When Joe was in his late teens, it became very difficult for his mom to care for him. So, his family arranged for him to move into a care facility. It seemed like a good idea at the time and Joe had high hopes of learning new skills while living in an environment much like the wonderful day school he had attended as a young child. It didn't turn out that way. Even though those ten years were a dark side of his life, because most of the other patients had severe developmental disabilities, he gained from this experience. He went through a special education program and earned his high school diploma.

The hardest thing Joe learned behind institution walls was that he would never learn to walk or speak clearly. Some, with his intelligence, were satisfied living in care facilities. But, knowing there was more to life and with a driving spirit to achieve the best life possible, he wasn't ever happy there.

At age twenty-seven, with the help of a good friend, Joe checked himself out of the first care facility. He then lived at a second facility for a few years and eventually got his own apartment through a subsidized program in the county where he lived. He has continued to live independently for over thirty years. He is currently in his mid sixties and lives in his own apartment in a complex dedicated to seniors and people with disabilities.

Finally living outside of institutions enabled Joe to attend college classes in writing. It also enabled him to publish the handicapped student newsletter at the college, meet people all over his community, have a girlfriend, hire and fire the people he required to take care of his needs, go on vacations with friends, pay his own bills, and manage his own life. Sometimes he gets into dangerous situations, has people take advantage of him, and even gets hurt occasionally. He considers all these things are just part of life.

Joe did enjoy a break from the pressures of living on his own when he lived with a friend for five years. They shared many of the decisions and problems that inevitably come up. Overall, they enjoyed a comfortable and pleasant life in his friend's home. There was a nice yard, a deck that he could sit on, birds to watch, her parents to visit in the mountains, and two dogs and a cat to play with and enjoy.

Joe has been a life-long learner and dedicated much of his time to bettering the lives of other disabled people. His parents, through the strength of their love and dedication, gave him the self-esteem to try everything and enjoy life. He hopes he has lived up to their dreams for what his life could be.

Joe has been writing poetry and short stories since he was about eleven years old. For many years, he wrote his poems on an old typewriter, using a crochet hook in his left hand, his good hand. His right hand is strong but not controllable. Fortunately, technology came along just in time. Through the generosity of one agency or another, he acquired a computer and then later another more advanced one. Special software programs enable him to use a stick with a curved point on one end to push in the keys one at a time through the holes in the plastic template positioned over the keyboard. The software program lets him have more than one key at a time pressed down, helps him find words, checks his spelling, and holds down the shift key for capitals and such.

In doing a word count of this book, he realized that he had entered over 200,000 characters and spaces into his computer one letter at a time, for the most part. The software does some word prediction for him, but he still has to enter many of the beginning letters of each word. That is an incredible number of times to place his hand on the keyboard template and move his hand around to get it into the correct position to hit the desired key. That number is amazing, even to Joe.

The word count above doesn't include the outlines for this book, Facebook entries, emails, short stories, blogging, and letters to the editor he wrote each day before and during work on this book. This is why he told somebody the two hundred words allowed in letters to the editor of the local newspaper are just a warm up for him.

This same computer that allows him to write also gives him a voice to communicate with the rest of the world. As only those who spend a great deal of time with him can understand his spoken word, especially on the phone, the computer has opened up the possibilities of communicating with people through on-line services, email, faxes, letters, essays, and even a voice simulator that can read to him what other people write.

Difficulty with other people understanding his speech hasn't kept him back. He received "The Communicator" award from the Dayle McIntosh Center for the Physically Disabled in southern California. He has been a life-long learner and dedicated much of his time to bettering the lives of other disabled people. He has based most of his short stories on living independently.

He can now send letters to the editors of newspapers, contribute articles to magazines, write a blog, comment on what other people write on the Internet, and share his essays, poems, short stories, and books with people all over the world. Joe is a happy man.

Nobody can make it alone, especially somebody who has cerebral palsy. Joe wouldn't be the man he is now, if he did not have the family he was part of and had not met and known some of the people he presents in this book. He wants to give credit to all the people who have helped him and made his life work. This book is his way of saying thank you to all of them.

October 8, 2010

People to Thank

Linda has done much of the proofing and given me insights on how to work my ideas into the narrative of the story. She is my right hand when it comes to editing and making things work together in the story. She helps me format my writing so that other people are able to read it and understand what I want to say. I would be lost without her help and this story would never have gotten to this point.

Mable knew I was going to throw away the idea for this story. It was just a part of another story, but Mable kept nagging at me to develop it into a story of its own. Every good writer needs somebody who nags.

Mr. Rooks has been more than just my teacher. He has been a motivator to keep me writing and working on this book. He is always telling me that I shouldn't go to the coffee bars and cafes as often as I do; instead, he says, I belong at home writing.

Mr. Good let me take his fiction writing class over as many times as the college would allow. He just told me to write one scene at a time and before I knew it, I had this book. He didn't realize how many scenes I would write. He was surprised when he kept seeing them come along in emails from me.

Mary believed in my writing way back and made me go to my first writing class.

The people who manage the apartment complex where I live give me a secure and safe home.

Scott helps me by adapting software and hardware so it works for me. Also, he keeps my computer operating smoothly and reliably. I am able to use it much more easily after he works on it. And he keeps it going and going. No matter what I do to mess it up, he fixes it.

Howard was working on his own book at the same time I was working on this book. We compared notes on our progress on a regular basis.

Jennifer was with me as a care provider for most of the writing of this book. She made sure I didn't have to worry about many of the little details of daily life.

Thank you to all of the people who have supported me in this project.

Joe Leroy Hemphill

Prologue

Prologue
By Frank, "The Gopher"

Hello good reader.

How are you?

Have you ever taken a creative writing class where the teacher told you to make your readers believe that something that never could happen really did? Well, I am Frank, the narrator of this story and I happen to be a gopher. Yes, you read that correctly, a gopher. You can say I am a cartoon character like Jiminy Cricket. That is okay with me, whatever works for you. Suspend your normal belief system, while reading this account, forget I am a gopher, and let Jerry's story unfold.

My father asked me to keep an eye on Jerry many years ago after my father couldn't do it any longer. I will explain why my father did that. When I first accepted this assignment, I had no idea how many people Jerry would meet and how many places he would take me.

A long, long time ago Jerry's grandfather saved my uncle, who was just a baby, by not flooding our family's tunnel. Jerry was just a baby too at that time. Because Jerry had cerebral palsy, he would need a great deal of watching over. So, after this event, my family took an oath to keep an eye on Jerry and help him if we could. Most parents will say that is the hardest thing to do, keeping an eye on a child while at the same time letting them be independent. So, we watched Jerry grow up and go through all the trials, dangers, hurts, and heartaches that everyone goes through.

Even after Jerry grew up, we still kept an eye on him. We could watch and do small things to help him. We could do things such as warning him about broken sidewalks, when he is out in his power wheelchair. We realized we could get in front of him and make him change directions to miss us. This was risky sometimes because Jerry might not see us and actually run over us. Luckily, that never happened.

Jerry has had cerebral palsy since birth but that is not why I found his life so interesting. He is handicapped and has done many great things but that isn't why others and I admire him. He would have done great things even if he weren't someone with a disability. It is the way he is made. Well, maybe I am getting ahead of myself.

My family never intended to share Jerry's story. We were just there to look out for him. But, in recent years, we all agreed that we needed to put it down in writing as it might help other families and individuals with cerebral palsy. And, since I received a new computer for Christmas, it became my project to write Jerry's story.

I feel as if I have gone back to school. I always believe in doing my research before I start a project. I found many notes from my grandfather and my father about Jerry and his family and all the other people in his life too. These helped to fill in the events that happened when Jerry and I were both very young.

Jerry had many people come in and out of his life. In his early years, they were mainly family members. Of course, there was his mom who had to be strong merely to get through all the everyday challenges and things that families face. Jerry's dad, who was around just long enough to give him a good beginning. His stepfather, whose behavior left a lot to be desired, was violent. We all, even gophers, have to deal with individuals we could live without. Jerry's stepfather was one of those.

After Jerry got older, his world expanded out past his family and he met many people. There was the lady who helped Jerry start to write a long time ago. And of course, there was George. George was the one who got Jerry started with his independent adult life. George was not sure Jerry would make it on his own.

Jerry has done much more than many people and George should get a great deal of credit for getting Jerry to a place where he would have the freedom to do these things. Of course, George also did some unusual things along the way. We all do but George was extraordinarily different. You will see what I mean as this story progresses.

Where should I start? Jerry's mom is a good place. She was there at the beginning and again later in his life. She helped make him who he is.

Ready?

Here goes.

Section One
Chapters 1 thru 6

Jerry, Age 0-17
Family

Section One - Chapter 1 - Jerry's Mom

Being Jerry's mom was not easy, to say the least. In 1943, when Jerry was born with cerebral palsy, there were no special programs for people with cerebral palsy. One doctor suggested sending Jerry away. Jerry's mom and dad decided to raise Jerry at home and give him as normal a life as possible.

Jerry only had his dad during his early years. But Jerry's mom and dad made good use of these early years to raise Jerry as normally as they knew how. Unfortunately, his dad died when Jerry was twelve and his brother Lance was eight, but at least Jerry and Lance had him in their lives for that long. Their mom then married a friend of the family who turned out to be abusive. So, these were rough years for the whole family and left very definite and lasting scars on Jerry, his mom, and his brother Lance.

Part of their idea for raising Jerry as normally as possible included Jerry doing chores. When Jerry was young, his mom made him mop the floor as one of his chores. Some neighbors thought Jerry's mom was heartless to have her son, who was disabled, mop floors. She would reply that she needed to treat her son the same as any other kid and that included him doing his chores. His mom didn't want him to think he was going to get special treatment just because he had a disability.

Back then, there were neither letter boards with the letters of the alphabet glued on them nor speech devices for communication. Jerry's dad and mom would rely heavily on Jerry's facial and body movements to understand him. One evening it took Jerry's dad an hour or more to understand Jerry's spoken words when Jerry asked for an allowance for doing chores.

All that Jerry wanted was that quarter at the end of the week for doing a good job mopping the floor. The only

problem Jerry had was keeping his brother Lance from
messing up the floor before his mom inspected it.

It was hard for his mom to see him go to a care facility
when he was seventeen. But it was the best and safest option
for him at the time. After Jerry went into the care facility, his
mom would write to him every week. This was how Jerry's
mom stayed in touch. But she didn't give Jerry a clue as to
what she and his brother Lance were going through with his
stepfather. Jerry thought everything was fine at home. It
wasn't until Jerry's twenty-first birthday that he found out just
how cruel and physically abusive his stepfather had been to
both Lance and their mom.

Except for visits back and forth, Jerry and his mom were
apart for about ten years, while Jerry lived in various care
facilities. Jerry went on with his own life, had girl friends, and
worked on his writing. Jerry also moved from one care facility
to another with help from a friend.

After ten years of living in care facilities, Jerry was among
the first group of people in the county with disabilities to move
out of a facility and into their own apartments. It was hard
going at times but Jerry never wanted to move back to a
facility.

After living on his own for a while, Jerry's life was calm
enough for him to attend college. He studied writing first at
Cypress City College and then at Long Beach State University.

Jerry was right in the middle of attending Long Beach
State University when his mom needed a place to stay and
asked to become his roommate and care provider. Jerry had
his doubts but agreed to the arrangement. It was hard for them
to get to know each other as adults and live together as
roommates.

Jerry and his mom had many battles about minor things
like what time Jerry should go to bed. All of Jerry's friends
now had to pass by his mom, who sat smoking in the living

room, before going back to Jerry's bedroom to visit him. If a girl stayed longer than Jerry's mom thought was acceptable, Jerry was asked many questions when the girl left. Jerry ignored these questions, went into his bedroom, and did homework or something.

There were times that Jerry and his mom enjoyed each other's company. They liked some of the same television shows but they watched them in separate rooms. Jerry's mom watched the TV in the living room and Jerry had a set in his bedroom.

His mom had her dog with her while she was living with Jerry. One day, while his mom was out, Jerry kicked the bedroom door to make the dog stop barking. Jerry was frightened that he had scared the dog to death, as it had suddenly grown quiet. He was afraid to face his mom because he thought he had caused the death of her dog. He was scared. He couldn't hide and didn't know whom to call. That dog meant everything to her. But luckily, the dog was okay.

Jerry liked doing small things for his mom, even though he would complain at the time. Every Tuesday, his mom insisted that he go buy three tabloid newspapers for her. Remember, this was before Jerry had a power wheelchair. So, he pushed his manual wheelchair backwards about a block to the store and then back again home just to buy her newspapers.

While getting his mom's newspapers at the store, Jerry didn't realize how much the tabloids would be a part of his writing. His mom encouraged him to write an article and submit it to the tabloids. So, to make his mom happy, one day he wrote a story for *The Star* newspaper and they wrote back asking him to answer some questions for the side bar that would go next to his article.

The teacher from Cypress City College helped Jerry write the answers to the questions for the side bar. The answers were what Jerry wrote about himself, as the writer, but from his mother's point of view and how she felt about him. About three weeks later, *The Star* printed his story and the side bar had his mother's name in it. Jerry got a check for $300.00 for his story. His mom was very proud. After that, Jerry didn't complain very much about going to get her newspapers for her.

For years, Jerry's mom carried articles with her that he had written and showed them to people she met. Some of these newspaper articles were turning brown because they had been in her pocketbook so long.

Jerry's mom always supported him, even when she was mad or upset with him. Jerry sometimes did things just to prove he could. And in Jerry's later years, he became very trying. The early power wheelchairs didn't have any breaking systems. This made driving one out on the street much more dangerous. Jerry made his mom walk behind him and watch while he drove his first power chair across the street.

When his mom moved out of his apartment, things were better between them. They decided to be friends and not boss and care provider. Jerry was no longer a little child who needed his mom to decide everything for him.

Jerry's mom didn't move very far away from him. She could have lived with her aunt, but the aunt lived a long distance from Jerry and Jerry's mom didn't want to be that far away from him. In a way, it merely went along with her promise to Jerry's father to take care of their son always.

Every week, when his mom came over to see him, he would ask her to do his laundry. Not all of it, but there were some special things that he wanted someone to handle with care. Jerry was surprised when his mom put out her hand for money. She wanted him to pay her just as he did everyone else who helped him. This wasn't a joke to her.

Over the next few years, they, on occasion would meet at a restaurant and have lunch together. Jerry always paid for these meals. Jerry became upset sometimes because his mom would take her meal home and not eat it while they were together. He didn't understand why she did this. It didn't dawn on Jerry until later that his mom was running short on money. The money that she had gotten from selling her home was almost gone.

Just before Easter, they went out for a nice meal and when his mom was walking to her car, she kind of lost her balance and hit a wall. This concerned Jerry. He knew something was wrong but wasn't sure what to do.

Then, three or four weeks or so later, at three o'clock in the morning, somebody called Jerry and told him his mom was in the hospital. Jerry called his aunt to tell her what was going on. She told him to get over to the hospital and that she was on her way. Jerry's aunt was really his great aunt and was very close to his mom. They were more like sisters.

Jerry got a neighbor to take him to the hospital and a male nurse bent down and told Jerry that his mom was very sick. Jerry went in to the room to see his mom. Her eyes were open and she looked at him and told him that she would be all right.

His mom smiled at him and then his neighbor asked her if she wanted someone to call her other son, Lance, to tell him what was happening. She said no, that she wanted her aunt to be there. By the time the hospital staff had taken his mom up to her room, she was no longer coherent and Jerry was never able to talk to her again.

Jerry did call his brother later that day. When Jerry's brother and aunt came to the hospital, they both pushed Jerry aside and took over the communication with the medical people. Jerry was there but not included in the decisions regarding his mother. Before they had arrived, Jerry had had everything under control. The nurses had come out to the waiting room every half hour and given Jerry an update on his mom. This stopped when his brother and aunt came and took control of the situation.

The doctors operated on his mother two different times. Jerry didn't try to stop them from doing any of these procedures because the doctors had given him a glimmer of hope that his mom might improve by undergoing the surgeries. In the back of his mind, he knew this was probably not the case. But, he agreed anyway.

His aunt would tell him that he would be to blame, if he didn't stop the procedures and his mom died. Jerry knew that was nonsense and didn't take it to heart. His aunt and brother didn't understand that the doctors would have had to operate anyway without any one saying yes or no. It was just a courtesy for them to ask his family. Jerry was the older brother and that is why they asked him.

One day, about a week after his mom got sick, Jerry asked his neighbor to take him over to the hospital before everybody else came. Jerry went in to his mom's room, said a prayer, then went over to the nurses' station, and gave them a note. Then all the people around the nurses' station listened while someone read his note aloud. His note said that he knew that his mom didn't want the doctors to bring her back to life if she would need life support. He thanked them for everything. Then he went home and never went back to the hospital. About a week later, just before Mother's Day, his mom died.

His mom had always wanted them to bury her next to Jerry's dad in Missouri. This is where they were from and where Jerry and Lance were born. So, Lance and Jerry's Aunt Ruth made all the arrangements. Even though things had gotten really dark at times just before Jerry's dad died, his mom and dad still loved each other very much. His dad always called his mom "Sug" which was short for "Sugar."

Some time later, Jerry asked a priest to say a special mass for his mom. Jerry thought the priest and he were alone in the church, but after the ceremony a lady from the back of the church came up to Jerry and said, "Your mom had a great son."

I am just a gopher but I agree with the lady. Jerry was a great son.

Section One - Chapter 2 - Jerry's Dad

Now I will talk about Jerry's father. Jerry's father was way beyond the current thinking, at the time, when it came to working with and doing things for children with disabilities. He had no training in doing this. He just naturally thought there should be better ways to do some things.

When his dad realized Jerry couldn't suck on a baby bottle like other babies, his dad cut a bigger hole in the nipple so more milk would come out. Then his dad would stay up all night putting a little bit of milk at a time into Jerry's mouth. One night, while doing this, his dad went to sleep and Jerry almost fell out of his lap.

In the mornings, Jerry's mom would take over giving Jerry milk while his dad went to work. They did this for several years until Jerry was big enough to drink out of a cup.

Jerry's dad was dedicated to the goal of making Jerry's life as normal as possible. This was obvious from the things he taught Jerry and how he treated him when he was a kid.

When Jerry was small, his dad put a big box in his room and bought him big stuffed animals to put in the box every night just to help him develop his coordination. Jerry didn't know then what his dad was trying to do. Jerry thought every body had a big box and put lots of stuffed animals and other toys in it. He remembered the animals were really big and he would walk on his knees to carry them to the box every night.

When Jerry was three or four, he saw his dad was wearing underwear with all kinds of colored stripes up and down. Jerry wanted to be like him. His dad told Jerry he would buy him underwear, if he learned to tell his mom when he needed to go to the bathroom. Also, he needed to get to the bathroom as quickly as possible so she could help him before he wet his pants.

At the time, Jerry had a baby walker. Their home had a big hallway and he made several marks on the walls of the hallway in his attempts to get to the bathroom in time. Somebody asked his dad why he let him wreck the wall and his dad said, "It's my wall and my boy." Then, about a month later, his dad bought Jerry underwear that looked just like the one's his dad wore. Jerry thought he was hot stuff. Every evening when his dad came home, his dad asked Jerry's mom if Jerry made it through the day without wetting his pants and she said, yes, he did.

His dad was a carpenter and back then they didn't have many toys for kids like Jerry. So his dad went out and built Lincoln log type blocks that Jerry could pick up and play with and try to put together.

His dad taught him all the numbers and how to tell time when Jerry was about five or six years old. His dad cut a piece of cardboard into a circle, wrote the numbers on it just like a clock, and added an arrow made out of cardboard that went around to all the numbers. He just had one arrow on the clock for a while.

At first, his dad would put the arrow at a different number each day and he would tell Jerry what number it was. After a while, he put another arrow on the clock and more numbers besides. Then every night he asked Jerry to tell him where the arrow was pointing. He talked to him and explained each number had five minutes between it and the next number. He worked with him for quite a while on the clock.

After working with the arrow and the clock for some time, Jerry's dad also worked on addition and subtraction with him. His dad would take Jerry out with him to work in the backyard. He would ask Jerry questions such as, "If a board is nine feet long, how many three-foot sections can be cut from it?" He would ask all sorts of questions like that while they were working. Jerry would think about them and then tell his dad the answers. When his dad took him to school the first time, Jerry's dad was very proud to show people what Jerry knew about telling time and numbers.

Jerry remembered his dad built a sandbox with legs on it. Kids at school were able to stand in a line next to the sandbox and play in it without actually having to get into the sandbox. It was a way for kids to get used to standing up in a secure situation. There was a brace or box built around each of them so they couldn't fall down. The box had a door with a latch on the back so the kids couldn't open it and fall out. The teacher at school would time each kid to see how long they could stand up on their own at the sandbox.

His dad never let Jerry use his handicap to get his way. One time his dad heard Jerry order his brother Lance to get a toy for him and his dad came in the room, picked Jerry up, and gave him a spank on his rear end. Not a bad one though. He just said, "You are able to get your own toy. Your brother is not your servant." Jerry was very surprised and he never did that again.

Another time Jerry's mom went out for the day and his dad was going to take care of him. Jerry asked his dad to take him outside to the backyard. His dad did that. Then Jerry asked his dad to take him inside the house. His dad did that. Then Jerry asked his dad to take him outside again. The next time his dad said, "Look, make up your mind or I will make it up for you." Then he whacked him on the butt and left him on the floor.

After that, Jerry thought before he asked anybody to take him somewhere. He learned to think about whether he really wanted to go and how long he wanted to be there. When his mom came home, his dad told her the new rule. That Jerry will only ask one time for someone to take him somewhere. His mom was very happy because she would get tired of taking him back and forth all day long.

His dad showed by example how to be kind to other people. He also taught Jerry not to take advantage of people and situations.

His dad showed Jerry how to listen to Lance and how not to be dependent upon Lance. He also showed him how to let Lance have his own life without Lance having to worry about him.

His dad bought Lance toys that his dad knew Jerry could never use or play with. His dad knew Lance needed to do everything, even if Jerry couldn't participate. His dad tried to teach Lance how to share by encouraging him to show Jerry how to play with the toys. Jerry enjoyed that. Jerry's dad hoped Lance and Jerry would be good brothers to each other.

Jerry always wondered if he had done what his dad had wanted him to do with his life and with Lance. Jerry didn't know what his dad had had in mind for him to be when he grew up. He hoped he had done what his dad had wanted and that his dad would be proud of him.

His dad had been very devoted to Jerry. He tried to give Jerry what he needed to be an independent person. He was just beginning to think of Jerry's future when he became ill from alcohol poisoning. His father had planned to be there when Jerry wanted to live by himself. There had already been talk of rooms Jerry's father was going to build behind the main house. Jerry would have been able to live by himself, or with that special lady, who may or may not have had disabilities. Jerry's father had seen a great future, even if he would have to build it himself for his son.

Jerry's father had tried not to groan when they lifted him on the gurney. But Jerry, at twelve years of age, had heard his father yelp like a hurt animal when they had to carry him from the bedroom through the small hall to the front room. Just before the paramedics had wheeled Jerry's father out the door to take him away to the hospital, his father had looked at Jerry and had said right to him, "Be a good boy and make me proud." All through Jerry's life, he didn't only try to be a good boy but also a good man.

I knew that Jerry had done what his dad had hoped for with his life, like being on the Board at United Cerebral Palsy. I wanted to tell Jerry that his dad, if he could see him now, would be very proud of him.

I thought Jerry was lucky to have had his dad for even the short time in his life that his dad was there. And he needed to remember what his dad had taught him. Jerry still misses his dad a lot.

Section One - Chapter 3 - Lance, Jerry's Brother

I couldn't ever get through to my brother Elmer about certain things. Elmer always wanted to use driftwood to brace every tunnel, because driftwood was light and easy to move. It didn't matter how many times I explained that driftwood wouldn't hold up very long. Elmer would persist in using it. Elmer never listened to me and always wondered why things didn't work out the way he wanted. Jerry had a similar problem with his younger brother Lance. It was hard to say whether Lance was naïve or he liked to make up his own reality.

When Lance started the first grade, he went over and asked another kid about the other kid's brother at home in a wheelchair. Lance thought everybody had a brother at home who used a wheelchair. At first, that early observation of Lance seemed to be cute but as they both grew older, Jerry saw that Lance was beginning to shape reality to fit what he wanted.

When Lance and Jerry were young, they had a typical relationship between two brothers. But, sometimes Lance would take advantage. Jerry had trouble with fine motor skills but, fortunately or unfortunately, he was good at math. Lance was always glad to break up their candy bars when their mother told them to divide one candy bar evenly between them. Often, Lance would try to convince Jerry that a Hershey bar only had nine squares instead of ten. Jerry knew he should have gotten five pieces of candy instead of four because he always got five pieces when their mom divided a Hershey bar. Jerry knew something was wrong. Lance always made up a reason for the missing piece. By some strange coincidence, the missing piece from Jerry's half always ended up in Lance's half. Their mom never caught on to what Lance was doing but Jerry did.

Jerry always told his mom to let Lance go out and play with the other kids. Even at a young age, Jerry didn't want Lance to lose out in doing something just because Jerry couldn't do it. When Lance came home, he would tell Jerry in detail what he did that day such as baseball, or tag, or whatever. So, Jerry got a feeling for how it was to go out and play in the neighborhood even though he couldn't actually go.

Overall, Jerry and Lance had a reasonably good childhood. Jerry remembered how they would spend hours at a time in their room putting a model together or playing chess. Lance liked to play the guitar in a neighborhood garage band. Jerry enjoyed going to Lance's band practices when Jerry came home from the care facility to visit his family for a few days.

The serious problems with Lance began when Lance was about sixteen years old and started having problems with substance abuse. Lance started lying to their mom about his friends and activities. One time, their mom bought Lance an electric organ for him to play his music on. She bought it on time and had to keep paying for it even after Lance had sold it for drug money. Their mom was working at a donut shop then and it took a long time to pay for that organ.

Jerry had to distance himself from Lance for Jerry's own safety. But, even then, Jerry always loved him. Lance was his brother. He's my brother; he's not heavy, as the song goes. I would sing this for you but I really am not a very good singer.

It broke Jerry's heart when he realized the direction Lance was going in. Jerry always tried to understand why Lance did this. Was it because Lance lost his real father at a young age? Was it because of their stepfather? Lance couldn't ever win approval from their stepfather no matter how hard he tried.

Jerry thought for a long time that, if he wasn't disabled, he might have kept Lance from drugs. But Jerry's friend convinced Jerry he really wasn't responsible for the choices

Lance had made. There are many reasons for people using drugs. It isn't for us to understand. We merely need to pray for people.

A few years after Jerry went to live in the care facility, he became very upset about everything that was happening there and asked them to call his mom. Jerry thought he just needed to talk to her. But, when Jerry heard his mom's voice, he realized just how unhappy he was and started crying. Lance got on the phone and said that he was on his way. Lance showed up about three hours later and they talked about why Jerry was so unhappy. Lance realized Jerry was upset about where Jerry was living.

While Lance was there, he talked with the administrator and tried to explain that Jerry needed more to do than just watch other people make crafts. Jerry couldn't control his hand movements well enough to do crafts himself. The administrator wouldn't listen to reason. The administrator said that he went to a lot of trouble to have a craft room and people there really enjoyed it, once they learned to make things. Lance could tell nothing would improve for Jerry by talking to the administrator. Since Jerry was late for dinner, Lance helped him eat. Soon after Lance left, Jerry did feel better because he had seen his brother.

Lance would have liked to have taken Jerry out of that place but things at home weren't going that well. Lance didn't tell Jerry about how their step dad was being mean to their mom. Jerry had enough to deal with living in that place. This was also during the time that Lance was getting more and more involved with drugs.

It was two or three years later when Jerry and Lance saw each other again. Lance served in the Navy during the Vietnam War. Jerry knew the name of the ship that Lance was serving on so he could listen to the news and follow the location of the ship and Lance. Lance also got married and had a baby during those years.

Some years later, with help from George, a friend, Jerry moved out of that place and a short time after that, he moved into his own apartment. This was when Lance came back into Jerry's life and tried to go back to his old habit of taking advantage of Jerry. This time it was worse than not dividing a candy bar evenly. Lance did something rather mean this time.

Lance brought a woman over to Jerry's apartment and had relations with her in the front room while Jerry was in the bedroom. Jerry was upset.

Jerry and Lance had been apart for so long that Lance hadn't prepared himself for how independent and tough Jerry was. So a few weeks later, Lance tried to do a similar thing, but this time, Jerry was ready. They went to the bar where Jerry was well known and Jerry asked a girl, who was his aide, to keep Lance busy for a while. The bartender helped Jerry go home and Jerry locked Lance out.

Lance had told their mom and his wife that he was going to take Jerry to the movies that night. Jerry put his radio on, went to bed, and cried into his pillow while Lance called him all kinds of names through the door. Lance finally gave up and called his cousin to take him in for the night. This wasn't the brother that Jerry remembered from their childhood.

It was a while before Lance and Jerry spoke again. Jerry was hurt about not being able to trust Lance. But, partly because Lance abused various substances, it was best for Jerry not to have Lance very involved in his life.

When Jerry was forty years old, he was lost for words when Lance made up a story about Jerry flying a jet plane, crashing, and ending up in a wheelchair. Jerry wondered what was wrong with saying that he had cerebral palsy and that even with that limitation he had become a successful writer. Jerry wouldn't have had any problem living up to that story. Jerry had never been in a jet and didn't have any desire to learn to fly. Jerry got into enough trouble just writing letters to the editor about political issues.

Years later, when Jerry moved in with a friend named Betty, she told Jerry he needed to reconnect with Lance. She could tell that it bothered Jerry that his brother didn't call or come around very often. They were still brothers and shared many memories. Jerry agreed and started to call Lance regularly. Jerry liked doing that and it seemed to fulfill a certain need inside of him. Jerry thought it would have pleased their mom too, if she were still alive.

Betty, and Mary Ann, another friend, took Jerry to visit Lance several times. Each time had been an unusual experience. Once they met Lance at a restaurant and Lance walked in sporting two cell phones. They were there almost two hours and Lance was on one or both cell phones most of the time. It seemed clear to Jerry that Lance still wasn't interested in learning about what was happening in Jerry's life. It was hard for Jerry to realize that Lance needed to be the center of attention all the time. This didn't leave any opportunity for Lance to learn about what Jerry was doing and accomplishing.

Lance had many business ventures over the years. One was a music shop and another was a non-alcoholic bar or nightclub. Lance was very excited about these businesses and wanted Jerry to visit and see him at work. Jerry didn't know why Lance wanted him to be there. Betty thought Lance wanted to show off to his older brother and make him proud. The sad thing about Lance has always been that he really didn't have to show off. He has always been very likeable and able to relate to many different people.

Lance has been married a number of times and has grown children, stepchildren, and grandchildren. Jerry knew or met all of Lance's wives and had been close to Lance's children when they were young. He really enjoyed playing with them and watching them grow up.

Recently, Jerry told Lance's daughter that nobody in the family knew who Jerry really was. The daughter told Lance what Jerry had said. This hit Lance very hard and made him really think about his relationship with Jerry. After that, Lance called Jerry almost every other day and came to spend Jerry's birthday with him. They worked to reconnect and share their lives with each other.

I was happy for Jerry and Lance. I decided to drop in and visit my brother Elmer. I brought him some Popsicle sticks to prop up his tunnels.

Section One - Chapter 4 - Hank, Jerry's Grandfather

I decided to take a day off from digging. Everybody needs days of rest and I should spend more time helping my family. Hank, Jerry's grandfather was a good example of someone who spent time helping his family. Jerry's grandfather showed Jerry how to be compassionate and how to comfort other people. He was 5'4", full-blooded Cherokee Indian, and a mean old goat.

When Jerry's dad passed away, his mom called Jerry's grandfather and he came as soon as possible. Jerry had the measles and the chicken pox at the same time, so he wasn't able to leave his darkened bedroom to go to his father's funeral. During this hard time, Jerry's grandfather brought him vanilla and orange sherbet ice cream. Jerry's grandfather would give Jerry a bite to eat and then ask him to guess which flavor the next bite would be. He made it a guessing game for Jerry to help distract him from what was going on and tried to let him know he wasn't alone.

During this time, Jerry could also hear his grandfather in the next room comforting Jerry's mom. His grandfather went back and forth between Jerry's mom and Jerry for about a week helping anyway possible. He didn't worry about anyone else for that week. Jerry's grandfather was just there for them. When his grandfather's wife would call, he would tell her that his job with the Indian tribe would have to wait longer than he first thought. For Jerry's grandfather, it was more important to be with his daughter and Jerry.

When Jerry's grandfather made up his mind to do something, he did it. For instance, when he decided Jerry needed some kind of wheeled chair to get around in. For the first twelve years of Jerry's life, Jerry didn't have any type of wheelchair. His mom and dad just hadn't given it much thought and perhaps in the back of their minds they hoped

Jerry, in time, would learn to walk some. Walking just wasn't in the picture for Jerry, even though he has tried several times over the years.

Up until that time, Jerry had moved about the house by rocking and scooting a small baby rocking chair back and forth from room to room. It took a lot of energy and a lot of time for him to go from room to room.

Jerry's grandfather asked Jerry's mom if it was okay for him to put wheels on Jerry's rocking chair. Jerry's mom said it was okay. The next day or the day after, his grandfather walked in with baby carriage wheels and two casters and he said to Jerry's step dad, "Come on I need you to hold it while I drill the holes." About half an hour later, Jerry's grandfather brought Jerry's chair back and put Jerry in it. Jerry went all over the house in no time. Lance was excited for Jerry and wanted a ride on Jerry's new, wheeled chair. Lance climbed on the back and Jerry went into their bedroom with him.

Jerry's step dad wasn't in favor of Jerry's chair having wheels on it. Jerry's step dad wasn't about to do anything for Jerry to make his life a little easier or give him some independence. Sorry, I am getting off track. Later, I will discuss Jerry's step dad, even though he wasn't worth the time of day. I just couldn't dig enough holes in the yard where he might step in one and break his neck. I tried and I tried.

Fortunately, Jerry's grandfather didn't pay any attention to Jerry's stepfather's objections and put wheels on Jerry's rocking chair anyway. Jerry's grandfather had taken an immediate dislike to Jerry's step dad and was glad to express his disapproval any time there was a chance. He even went out of his way to cause incidents where he could voice his opinion. No, he definitely wasn't the shy and retiring type.

Jerry's grandfather had an unusual sense of humor. He would go to the other room as if he was going to the bathroom or something. Then he would come back and put his hands on the table and one finger would be all beat up. It was a rubber finger. Or, he would stand next to a table and put his hand down as if he was going to talk to you about something else. Meanwhile you look down and you see this awful bloody finger.

Jerry's grandfather had several other tricks too. One time, Lance brought over a girl for the family to meet. Jerry's grandfather went into the bedroom, put Jerry's mom's high heels and wig on, and then came out to meet Lance's friend. Lance went down the room introducing everyone and saying, "This is my brother and this is my mom." Lance looked at Jerry's grandfather at the end of the room and he didn't know what to say. It took Lance a few seconds to get over how his grandfather looked. But after examining the situation, Lance continued with introducing his new girlfriend to everybody. It wasn't everyone who had a grandfather who wore high heals. Lance wondered how he got so lucky.

Jerry's mom said, "Daddy don't do that." Lance thought that Jerry was supposed to be the problem he had to deal with but the grandfather was the one.

Fortunately or unfortunately, Jerry picked up on the same weird type of humor as his grandfather. Sometimes, when a person asked Jerry to go get something, he would simply reply that he didn't walk. Jerry usually caught people off guard and he would merely smile. Jerry's humor got him through some difficult situations. Once his step dad hurt his leg and he was in extreme pain. Jerry rolled past and calmly suggested the leg could be cut off up near the groin. Jerry's step dad was in too much pain to move. Jerry just wheeled into the bedroom. Mark one up for Jerry.

Jerry's grandfather had a habit of wearing a hat everywhere he went. It was either a brown or a black Indiana Jones style hat. When his grandfather ate, he wore it. When his grandfather talked to people, he wore it. Everywhere his grandfather went, he wore his hat. Many years later, Jerry unconsciously took up wearing a similar hat. If Jerry's grandfather had been there, he would have smiled to see a younger version of himself in Jerry. I think he would have been so proud of his grandson, Jerry, and all of Jerry's accomplishments.

Section One - Chapter 5 - Stu, Jerry's Stepfather

I have mentioned Jerry's step dad before. Jerry's real father had had so many great ideas and plans for when Jerry got older. His father had wanted Jerry to be independent and strong. Things turned out very different for Jerry, mostly because his step dad took control of the whole situation. And the guy was cruel, conniving, and an all around despicable person. My whole family and I disliked that poor excuse for a human being.

That good-for-nothing named Stu came into Jerry's life at probably the worst possible time. Jerry's real father had just passed away and Stu had been right there and immediately moved in to take advantage of the situation. Earlier on the day that Jerry's dad had died, Jerry had watched the paramedics take his father away. Jerry was terribly upset that entire day. When they told Jerry that his father had passed on, Stu slept next to Jerry to comfort him. Jerry had thought Stu was a nice guy at this point.

Stu moved in on Jerry's mom the same way. He acted like a nice guy. Stu had been a friend of Jerry's father. Jerry's mother didn't know exactly how she was going to raise two kids alone. His mother knew there were going to be many problems to face while Jerry was growing up. For that reason, at the time, Jerry's mother was glad to have Stu there. He seemed like a nice guy at first, for about a year.

Then things changed for no apparent reason. Stu did mean and cruel things to Jerry and his brother Lance. Years later, Jerry started telling people what had happened. I don't think Jerry could have made all this up. If people, at the time, had heard these stories about Stu, they would have thought Jerry had made them up, but friends, Jerry wasn't that good of a liar. Besides, Jerry's Aunt Ruth and his grandfather Hank had picked up on the real Stu at the very beginning. They both didn't trust him or his motives for moving in so quickly on this very vulnerable family.

To the outside world, Stu was that great man who stepped in after Jerry's father died and took care of this small woman with two kids, including one with disabilities. What a great guy. Great guy? Yeah, my grandfather wished he could have poured sewer water down Stu's mouth. That was what Stu needed. But, like Jerry, my grandfather couldn't do much to defend Jerry and his family or to retaliate. They all just had to endure.

Stu would be mean to Jerry sometimes for no reason at all. Stu was a postman and could come by the house anytime. Stu would come home throughout the day on the excuse of helping Jerry in the restroom. Jerry's mother would take Jerry earlier to keep him from having any unnecessary contact with Stu. Stu would walk by and thump the top of Jerry's head with two knuckles. Jerry already had brain damage from cerebral palsy so why not do more damage. Who would even know? Jerry's mother tried to come to Jerry's rescue but Stu did this so quickly she didn't have a chance to catch him. Lance tried to get Jerry into the bedroom whenever he could and away from Stu.

Jerry also had a reading problem. He couldn't remember what he read so therapists and teachers encouraged Jerry to read aloud to improve his retention of what he read. Stu, the candidate for cruel jerk of the century, made fun of him when Jerry would read aloud alone in his room.

Today, people are amazed that Jerry cannot really read, because he writes so well. Please, I say again please, don't tell Jerry he writes well. Every time somebody tells Jerry he is a good writer, he acts odd, and thinks he is the best thing since sliced bread. His care provider can't spend time taking care of him because she has to listen as he explains in detail how far he has come in his writing. He will even go back twenty years explaining how he wrote for the university newsletter and how he did it all on an electric typewriter. That may be great and all. But his poor care provider has to sit there with a spoon of oatmeal held in mid air as he tells the same story for the tenth time. Jerry doesn't know how close he has come to getting oatmeal thrown in his face.

The meanest thing Stu did was the day Stu took Jerry outside and washed him like a dog with the hose because Jerry needed a bath. Jerry was about 12 years old when this happened.

Another incident happened when everyone at the day school went swimming. Jerry had forgotten to remind a mentally challenged boy, who had helped him change into his swimming trunks earlier, to bring Jerry's blue jeans to the pool. So, when Jerry got out of the pool, he didn't have his jeans to wear home. He only had his underwear. People at the day program made sure Jerry had something covering him while the taxi took him home.

Everything was good until the taxi drove up into Jerry's driveway. Then Stu came out of the house, proceeded to remove the towel, and held Jerry upright, making him walk from the taxi across the yard and in the front door. Jerry knew all the neighbors could see him in his underwear. You could say Jerry was among the first streakers. He was always ahead of his time. Ahead of his time or not, he was very embarrassed and humiliated at being forced to do that. Jerry was maybe fourteen when that incident happened.

I am sure my grandfather wanted to chew Stu's feet off. Look, Jerry was struggling with the idea of becoming a man. He certainly didn't want to parade around in the yard with just his underwear on. Jerry was already having trouble with the idea of his mother dressing him every day.

Sometime later Jerry wanted to get back at Stu. Jerry had had enough. But what could he do. After much thought, Jerry decided he would just stare at Stu. When Stu watched TV, Jerry looked at him. When Stu ate dinner, Jerry looked at him. When Stu was reading, Jerry looked at him. Even when Stu was sleeping, Jerry looked at him. Jerry met Stu at the door in the evening when he came home from work, so he could look at Stu. Jerry didn't say a word. He just looked at Stu. After two weeks, Jerry decided he had better things to do and Lance was glad to have Jerry back to play with him and help build his model airplanes.

When Jerry was seventeen, he knew he was taking a lot of his mother's time with what he needed in care. And, Jerry's mother really wanted to get Jerry away from Stu before Stu really hurt Jerry. Stu was beginning to be more open about abusing Lance and Jerry. Stu was the main reason for Jerry's mom sending Jerry to live in a care facility but Jerry didn't know that until much later.

Jerry thought he was going to a place where he would receive more training as he had in the day program. He was actually kind of excited about going away to school. Jerry sure was wrong about that one. Jerry just went from one bad situation to another. Who knew? The booklet and pamphlet looked good. And Jerry's mother was running out of time and ideas.

Jerry's mom had promised Jerry's real father she would take care of their sons. A few years after Jerry was out of the house, Lance joined the Navy at sixteen. His mother signed the forms because she thought it would be better and safer for Lance in the Navy than at home with Stu.

Jerry had thought things would get better for his mother if he wasn't there. Going away to live at the care facility seemed to solve the problem. Lance wanted things to be better for his mother too and the Navy seemed like the perfect idea to get him out of the house. They could not have known that things could and did get worse for their mother after they both left the house.

Jerry didn't know what was going on at home during those years after he went away to the care facility. Then his mother and his Aunt Ruth came to see him on his twenty-first birthday. This was when they told Jerry that Stu had beaten Jerry's mother so severely it put her in the hospital. Also, because of that, Stu was gone. Jerry's Aunt Ruth had insisted to his mother that his mother needed to tell Jerry what had happened. This was not a pretty picture for him to digest on his twenty-first birthday. After his family left, Jerry went outside behind the "jail house," as he often referred to the care facility, and softly cried all through that eerie evening. Happy Birthday, he thought to himself through his tears.

Section One - Chapter 6 - Jerry's Aunt Ruth and Two Uncles

Most families have one person that everybody goes to in troubled times or just when they need to talk to someone. In Jerry's family, it was his Aunt Ruth. Like everyone else in Jerry's family, his Aunt Ruth didn't see the need for anyone to treat Jerry differently. He was a kid and all kids needed toys and crayons. She just found things that would work better for him.

His aunt looked all over for large-scale coloring books for Jerry to use at home and at school. She bought him large crayons that didn't break easily, too. Who knew this activity, using crayons, would later on help Jerry to learn to hold his typing stick? In many ways, Jerry's whole family did things that were beneficial for his physical development. It was hard to say whether they planned it that way or they just wanted to try everything they could think of that might help Jerry. It certainly was not for a gopher to say. I had enough trouble building and maintaining tunnels. They were mainly trying to allow him to experience as many typical kid activities as possible.

Jerry's aunt was married to a guy named Tom, when Jerry was little. Tom would come to the house, pick up Jerry, and take him to the stables. Aunt Ruth and Uncle Tom boarded their horse there. Uncle Tom would put Jerry on the horse and Jerry would ride all morning. That was a way for Jerry to learn to keep his balance. Because he had developed his balance by riding their horse, no one had to tie him into a chair like many with cerebral palsy. His uncle would hide behind a hill and Jerry would feel as if he was alone out on the range looking for cattle.

Jerry's uncle died when Jerry was about sixteen and his aunt married a guy named Paul. Jerry's new Uncle, Paul, built freeways for the state.

One day, Jerry was in his apartment and heard hammering. When he looked out his front door, there was Uncle Paul building a ramp for Jerry's wheelchair. His uncle got up off his knees and stood back. He looked it over and said "not bad but the union may come and inspect it."

For a while, every Friday, his uncle would look up at the clock and say its time for Jerry to call and Jerry would. It seemed that Jerry's power wheelchair would break down and his uncle would come and take it to the wheelchair company to get it fixed.

One time, Jerry's brother, Lance, left dope in Jerry's apartment and Jerry called his aunt and asked her what he should do with it. She told him to flush it down the toilet, and he did. When his brother came back and asked what happened to his stash, Jerry just smiled and told him it was in the toilet. Lance's eyes got big and he walked out.

Sometimes, Jerry needed some extra money. He would call his aunt and she would say this was just a loan. But he and his aunt knew he couldn't pay it back.

Jerry was in the car with his aunt one day. He was surprised when she suddenly pulled over, turned up the radio, and started shouting at the horse race. She had obviously placed a bet on it. Then Jerry knew where all of the extra cash from his aunt was coming from.

It was later in Jerry's life when his aunt played a more prominent role concerning him. When he did not want his mom to know something, like when he went out drinking or he wanted a woman, he would call his aunt and talk about things. He always asked her not to tell his mom. Everyone needs someone who will just listen and not judge. For Jerry, it was his aunt. When he did something wrong, his aunt would talk to him like a grownup and not like a child.

There was the time Jerry went with his aunt to buy a refrigerator. His aunt made sure that the salesperson talked directly to him and not to her about the refrigerator. She also set it up where he could make the payments. But when Jerry went back to get the refrigerator they refused to let him pay for it in installments. So his aunt went down and paid for the refrigerator and he made payments to his aunt every month.

One afternoon, his aunt wanted to get away from all her problems with some of the other members of her family and she asked Jerry to meet her at a restaurant. They had a good time. His aunt was able to relax and tell him everything that was bothering her.

Jerry learned from his uncles and aunt how to handle himself out in the world. His aunt and both uncles taught him how to enjoy life while also taking responsibility for his actions.

Section Two
Chapters 7 thru 12

Jerry, Age 17-30
Care Facilities

Section Two - Chapter 7 - Sam, Jerry's Roommate

I was finishing a sand wall in a tunnel, when Jerry met Sam. Only a well-skilled gopher like me can work with sand. You need to be fast and exact or sand won't stay in place long enough to construct another wall. I have had a six-room cave built before a high tide rolled up. Well, enough about my problems. Jerry, about this time, met Sam. Jerry and Sam would become good friends but the start was somewhat rocky.

In the beginning, Jerry was not quite sure about Sam. Most of the other "inmates" or residents were short on the smarts and Jerry wasn't too sure about the new guy. It took almost six months for them to say, "Hello." to each other. Jerry noticed Sam was always reading news or sports magazines. That wasn't normal behavior in that place. Sam wasn't too sure about that guy Jerry, who spent most of his time working on an electric typewriter. It surely didn't take him that long to learn the alphabet. But in time, they discovered that they both were all right and became great friends.

They both lived in that residential facility for many years and became roommates too. It was sometime, however, before these two became roommates and it wasn't under the best of circumstances. Jerry had been home visiting with his family for a few days. On his return, he learned that one of his best friends had passed away suddenly. Before his friend had died, the facility had moved all of Jerry's personal belongings into his friend's room, where Sam lived too. Sam told Jerry that their friend, who had died suddenly, had told Sam, the day before their friend died, that he was glad Jerry was going to be in their room because the three of them had a lot in common.

Sam explained to Jerry how all this had come about. Two other guys, who had been in that room with Sam and their friend who died, had gotten into a fight. The administration decided to separate the two guys by switching one of them with Jerry. So they moved all of Jerry's things into the other room and they moved one guy's belongings into Jerry's old room.

A week later, after all the moves and their friend had died suddenly, the hospital then moved both Sam and Jerry into a different room with two mentally retarded guys. This unexpected change thrust Sam and Jerry into the daily battle not to lose their minds. One of the guys in this new room had a TV and changed the station every two minutes. The other guy merely talked to himself and his imaginary friends. Jerry soon learned the names of all the people and animals that were part of this guy's make believe world. Sam became concerned about him when it looked as if Jerry had joined their roommate in his make believe world. Jerry assured Sam everything was all right and it was just a game.

They both wanted to do the right thing about one of the guys that the aides always picked on. They felt protective towards him. They tried yelling at one of the mean aides, but it didn't do much good. They both realized there probably wasn't much they could do about it. It still bothered both of them though.

Sam watched the nightly news on television and he got Jerry into the habit of watching the news too. They both followed the Vietnam War. When word came out about the death of President Kennedy, Jerry searched for Sam all through the building. Jerry peered into Sam's eyes for some answer. There wasn't any. Then there was the morning that Jerry woke up and Sam had told him that someone had shot and killed Robert Kennedy. Jerry said that isn't funny. Sam just agreed.

Sam followed sports, especially the local community college team. Jerry thought Sam was foolish to follow sports.

When Sam got involved with the boosters club, Jerry told him he wasn't going to go anywhere with it.

Sam thought Jerry was a good writer. But, he also thought Jerry needed to cooperate more with the management where they lived. In order to be able to write, Jerry needed a place set up for his typewriter where he could work undisturbed. When the management wanted to punish Jerry, they took away this access to his typewriter.

Sam went on to be a success at writing about sports while still living at the facility long after Jerry left and also on the outside many years later. Every year he won an award. He became the historian for not only the baseball team but also for the whole sports department at the college. Jerry is still jealous and happy for him at the same time. Jerry went on to be a successful writer after he moved away from the facility.

They both found success but really only talk to each other once a year or so. It sill bothers Jerry that they are not close anymore. His friends have told Jerry that it is all right, as he and Sam had been close friends and did have a good time for a number of years. They both learned from each other and supported one another in following their dreams.

Section Two - Chapter 8 - Diane, Activity Director

Diane came to work in the residential facility where Jerry and Sam were living. The institution hired her to help the people who lived there learn to read and write or whatever else they needed help with. She arranged classes and helped people individually with life skills.

Diane met Jerry one day and asked him what he was doing. He answered that he wasn't doing anything. Jerry had just completed all the graduation requirements for high school. Like many people just out of high school, he really didn't know what he was going to do. The hospital didn't have any programs or activities that really interested him. He wasn't able to do crafts as most people living there spent their time doing.

Living at what he called "the jail" put some limitations on looking for employment. He knew there were jobs and other opportunities that he was missing but right then he couldn't change the situation. His cerebral palsy ruled out being a surgeon. This was one of Jerry's jokes about his situation. I won't labor you with the other ones.

He had written a little bit way back in the day program when he was young and in high school. But, he really didn't take it seriously. It was in a training school where he had learned to type holding a stick in his left hand and hitting keys through holes in a plastic template that was over the keyboard. In Jerry's jail, he had a typewriter and a nurse had given him a little closet where only a desk and a small table would fit. He could work on his typewriter in this closet.

So, when Diane asked him what he might like to do, he told her he was a little interested in writing. Before he knew it, Diane had a book about writing out and every week she would read a part of the book to him. Diane would give him homework assignments to write stories using the information from what she was reading. Then, she would go over the stories he wrote and make corrections and suggestions.

Diane went all through that book with him. Each part was about an aspect of writing such as plot or scene. After each assignment, he would type out the main points of each chapter and put them in a little brown notebook that she had given him. Many years later, he had someone retype the notebook and put all those notes in his computer. Over the years, he wore out that little notebook going through it to refresh his understanding of terminology and different aspects of writing. When he went to college at Cypress and then at Long Beach, anytime he didn't understand something in a class, he would go back to that little notebook that Diane helped him create.

One of the stories he wrote during this time was good and a national rehabilitation magazine contacted him regarding publishing it. Somebody called the local newspaper and they did a number of stories about him, his typewriter, and the story he was working on for the magazine. The guy from the paper wrote an article based on each correspondence from the magazine detailing what Jerry went through while he re-wrote his story or responded to the magazine editor. The magazine finally published Jerry's story. And, the newspaper wrote a wrap up on what was involved in getting his story edited and ready to publish. They focused on how somebody like Jerry, with cerebral palsy, had published a story in a national magazine.

But his successes were stopped by the institution, sorry to say. The head nurse, who had given him the closet, was no longer in favor with the owner. So, the people in control moved his typewriter into the library where everybody worked on things like math and reading. That was the end of the road for developing a special skill in that place. The hospital administrator, or the head jailer, as Jerry would have said, believed everybody there should just do crafts. This was just one of the many things where Jerry and the administrator didn't agree.

Diane taught him much more than writing. She taught him that, if you believe in something, you had to go out and do it.

Not long after his story was published, Diane was fired because she was becoming too involved with one of the "inmates," him. Jerry was in contact with her for a while after she left. She even came over to his mom's house one time when he was there for a visit.

Diane helped many people besides Jerry. Jerry had originally thought they hired Diane to help people like himself, who wanted to learn new things. Actually, they just wanted her to keep everybody occupied not so much really learning anything new. Before moving to that facility, his mom and he thought he could learn and improve himself while there.

Jerry sometimes has to remind himself that he had people who were supportive at the beginning of his writing career. He has Diane to thank for being the first one who recognized his ability and encouraged him to pursue writing.

And today, when his articles appear all over the world via the Internet, he realizes he has had people like Diane who came into his life, pushed him, and helped him to keep pursuing writing, which has become his life's goal and crusade. He didn't do it alone, Diane was right there beside him when he made the discovery that writing was what he really wanted to do with his life.

He wishes that Diane could have known how he continued with writing long after she was no longer guiding him. He secretly smiles at the idea that Diane might have come across his work, read it, and known that she was instrumental in encouraging him to pursue what has turned out to be his life-long passion. He really hopes that Diane had a good life and got to spend her time helping other people discover their talents, passions, and abilities. It was obvious to him at the time that her passion was helping other people find theirs.

Section Two - Chapter 9 - Kay, Jerry's Friend

Jerry didn't realize what an emotional roller coaster Kay was going to be. Like Jerry, I had thought Kay was going be good for Jerry. It seemed he had finally found a lady to be with but it surely didn't turn out to be that way. He first met Kay in the "jailhouse" care facility where they were both living.

At night, Jerry would eat his nightly snack of cheese crackers. The staff scattered the cheese crackers on a towel that they had spread across the table. By putting his mouth down to the table, he was able to grab them with his teeth. He always made a mess but nobody really complained. Eating cheese crackers at night was one of the few times when he could eat something on his own and not need anyone else around. He could just have a quiet time to think and contemplate.

He liked his roommate Sam, but Sam was almost the only one Jerry could carry on a conversation with. The other patients had a wide range of developmental disabilities and thus talking with them was hard.

One night, while eating his crackers, Jerry looked up and Kay was in the hall and getting a Coke from the machine. Kay was also in a wheelchair. He watched her for a while. He decided that, if she was able to do that much, the girl wasn't retarded like most of the other residents.

Many times after that night, Kay joked that she was glad she had passed the test of getting her own soda. Kay told Jerry later that she had thought he was a genius because he was typing all the time. So these were the reasons they had not talked with each other while living almost a year in the same place. Every evening after dinner, Jerry went with Kay back to the dining room or outside on the patio and they would read or talk.

Jerry didn't waste any time when he realized he had a live one on the line. After a month, they started meeting a second time every night around eleven in the dining room. They kissed and hugged each other. Yes, in deed, they became lovers. Unfortunately, there were rules against this in the place where they lived. They had to be careful when and how they showed affection.

For a while, every morning, Jerry would go outside, pick a rose, and bring it back for Kay. She really liked the gesture, put the rose in her lap, and then put it in her room in a special vase. Everything seemed to be going well for Kay and Jerry.

Jerry's mom helped him buy a bathrobe for Kay's birthday. His mom acted as if she didn't know why he insisted that the robe had to have snaps to secure it instead of buttons or a zipper. He was always thinking ahead. Kay wore it many times.

But, then one night the nurse caught Kay and Jerry hugging and kissing in the dining room and talked to them as if the were children. The nurse then asked them what they would do if a baby came. This seemed like a dumb question to them. They looked at each other and thought how they were sitting in their wheelchairs, not on the floor. They let the nurse go through her routine without reacting and agreed not to do it any more. They just found another place to go to be alone. Some people working at that place just couldn't understand about how and why Jerry and Kay needed to be together.

Each Sunday Jerry would watch people from many churches come. He felt more alone on that day so he decided to reach out. He knew deep inside he needed more than just his writing to make his life fulfilling and complete. He started attending the various services that local churches provided at the care facility. The priest from a local Catholic Church came to where they lived also and said Mass for the residents. Jerry realized the Catholic services appealed to him more than the others. He also noticed that Kay was more at peace with herself after attending the Catholic Mass.

So, Jerry started attending the Catholic Church services on a regular basis with Kay. After attending these services for a while, Jerry decided he wanted to have himself baptized as a Catholic. Some people thought Jerry did this only to be with Kay. Even being a gopher, I could tell that was nonsense.

There was no great enlightening that came over Jerry. He just decided to do something and then did it. That was how Jerry did most things. Whatever thoughts he might have about the consequences of his actions would come long after doing something. He would then try to figure out how to get out of whatever he had done. But that wasn't the case when he became a Catholic.

The priest came to see Jerry to find out if he truly wanted to become a Catholic. This first time he came, Kay helped the priest to understand Jerry's speech and explained how to use his letter board. After that, Jerry would also write notes for the priest, if Jerry needed something answered. The priest came to the care facility every week to talk to Jerry and read from a Catechism book. This went on for at least six months.

For a long time, Kay would read to Jerry about different saints. And they would talk about what they were reading. But, when Jerry had asked a priest to get him ready for baptism, Kay tried not to read anything that the priest might have been discussing. Kay didn't want to confuse Jerry or influence him.

One night, Jerry was very upset because somebody in the care facility got mad at Jerry's long hair, so the priest and Kay talked to Jerry for a while. It was more important than the lessons that night to let Jerry get out his frustration. Jerry and Kay wondered if the priest went home with a headache that evening.

There were still people who thought Jerry was becoming a Catholic just because he wanted to be with Kay but that wasn't the case. They both made sure it was what Jerry really wanted to do.

When it was time for Jerry's baptism, most everybody from the care facility came to watch the ceremony. Some people even brought presents for Jerry.

Eventually, sometime later, it became apparent to Jerry that Kay had developed a mental problem or maybe always had had one. Kay started telling him that her problems stemmed from her relationship with her mother. Kay was always trying to please her mother and it was obvious to everybody watching that she would never be able to do it. Jerry went off his rocker trying to help Kay during that time when they were so close. Sometime later, Jerry had to go to a psychologist about what he was feeling and going through with Kay.

Because of the lack of freedom, it became very important that Jerry and Kay find another place to live. Kay's mother found the new place that was a hundred and fifty miles away from where they had met and lived for many years. Kay's mother lived near the new facility and helped Kay move there. Jerry's friend George helped Jerry move.

At the new facility, they had more freedom and became lovers again. Kay was always there when somebody didn't understand Jerry's speech. Jerry was always there when Kay got upset about her mother. Jerry was still troubled about Kay and her problems. This didn't change in the new facility. He still loved her but it was getting increasingly difficult to deal with her instability.

In the new place, Jerry and Kay could stay up as late as they wanted. One night Kay told Jerry that he didn't have to go find someone to undue his pants so he could get undressed when he wanted to go to bed. She could do it for him. Kay was about to undue Jerry's pants one night, just when the nurse walked by, saw them, and kept on going. But the next day, the nurse, a guy, just had to say something cute to them. He said, "You want me to believe that Kay was just helping you undue your pants?" We said it wasn't what it looked like. Occasionally, the nurse, with a smile, would ask Jerry about his pants. Jerry would just shake his head and laugh.

Jerry and Kay were in that place for about two years before they moved out. A social worker decided Jerry should be one of the first persons with a disability to live outside of an institution. Some other people like Jerry also moved into their own apartments and that trial arrangement was a big success. So, today, thousands of people live the same as Jerry does, in their own apartments. Jerry also manages three or four care providers at a time who often become his close friends.

At the same time Jerry moved into his own apartment, Kay moved back home with her mother. About six months after moving in with her mother, Kay moved into her own apartment too. She tried it for a few years but it never worked out very well for her. Jerry tried to help her adjust to living on her own. But, Kay never could adjust to living outside of an institution. That was odd because she didn't have as involved physical disabilities as some people including Jerry. But she did have deep emotional issues that Jerry couldn't handle any longer. Sometimes she wanted Jerry to be a lover and other times her brother. She would change these roles on him without any warning.

After they moved out of the institution, Kay and Jerry talked on the phone on a regular basis. Kay took over his life by wanting him to come to her with every problem and she wanted to tell him all her problems every day. Jerry got tired of their conversations being centered around her problems with her mom and other people. She didn't know how to relate to people. She would make up outlandish scenarios for why people were doing really quite innocent things.

Kay was so psychologically and emotionally unstable that Jerry realized he didn't want to continue the relationship any longer. He wanted to get on with going to school, meeting new people, and having a normal life now that he was outside of the care facility. Kay still couldn't adjust to life outside of the care institution and all the relationships and interactions involved.

Kay's instability had affected Jerry's life for many years and her grasp on reality was deteriorating rapidly. He realized he couldn't help her with her problems and she was causing him great stress and emotional turmoil. So Jerry had to tell Kay not to call him anymore with all of her problems. He was very sad about how their relationship was ending.

They did talk and see each other occasionally after this, but Kay became even more unstable. Jerry finally had to brake off completely all communication with her. It was the only way for him to keep his own sanity.

Some years later, I came across some information that shed more light on what should have been a wonderful relationship for Jerry and Kay. Did you know a gopher could work a computer? I learned from watching Jerry. And one day I was looking for a database file in Jerry's computer and found a letter he had written Kay. He never sent it. It is interesting. Here, I will read it to you. Jerry won't mind. Hey, he won't even know.

. . . .

Dear Kay,

I'm not saying you didn't help me when we first met. You gave me someone to care about besides myself when we were in the institution. I remember how we met in the dining room after all the patients were in bed and the nurses were busy with reports. Man, could we make out!

As I think about it now, the best times we had were inside an institution. Yet our goal was to move out of institutional life and live in an apartment. I did it but you couldn't handle it. You could speak better than I could and you had much better control in your arms and hands. But something inside just wouldn't allow you to be free!

I know your mother had a great influence over you. She had many psychological problems. Or maybe she didn't. Sometimes I wondered if you had more psychological problems than your mother did. I don't know. But I do know I didn't need to go to a psychologist before I met you.

It doesn't matter whether you're handicapped or not, there comes a time when you have to tell your mother that you want to move out on your own and handle your own life. You talked a lot to others about doing this. But you never truly did it yourself!

I'm not blaming you for any of my problems. It was my fault that I allowed you to have such an influence in my life. I should have known when to shut you out of my life. But I still loved you for a long time.

Jerry

Section Two - Chapter 10 - George, Jerry's Friend

Jerry had asked his former high school teacher if she knew anyone who could help proof his stories. In about two weeks, George showed up. George was only fifteen at the time and his mom brought him every Saturday for two hours or so. I was building my living room when George entered Jerry's life. George was an eccentric, interesting, and strange character. I put aside my work to study George.

For example: the first two times Jerry met with him, George would pick up Jerry's typewriter and carry it to wherever they went because George didn't understand Jerry and needed him to type out what he was saying. Most people could learn to understand the way Jerry spoke in a little while but George needed more time. For about two months, George carried Jerry's typewriter from room to room so they could communicate.

Later on, George began to understand Jerry's speech. They talked about many things and became good friends. At the time, Jerry had no idea that George was going to help him change his life forever. Probably, if either of them had realized what the future held, they both would have run away from each other. But, it was the sixties and they both were eager for adventure.

When the care facility became unbearable for Jerry, George began to look around for some place else for Jerry to live. At one time, George wrote a letter to a care facility in Arizona. A religious order ran the institution and, at the time, Jerry was more religious. The only thing they got back was a stack of prayer cards and some seeds. Soon, the two adventurers became disheartened with this plan of attack. The prayer cards were nice but Jerry was still in a place where he really didn't want to be.

While our two heroes were thinking of what to do next, Kay's mother told George and Jerry about this place in Torrance where it would be better for Kay and Jerry. By that time, the jailhouse had become more controlling about who could take the inmates out. George and Jerry had to secretly plot and make long-range plans in order for Jerry just to go to see the new place. Every week, George would come by and take Jerry for a ride for an hour or two. Then, when the people in charge got used to them going out once a week, George made an appointment to see the other place and they didn't come back for about eight hours.

As it usually happened on their outings, something went wrong. George's car ran out of gas and he had to walk to a gas station and come back with gas. That made the outing even longer. The people that ran the jailhouse were not pleased that they were so late getting back.

When the care facility found out what Jerry and George had been up to, they were really upset and mad. They made it difficult for Jerry and George. They didn't trust George any longer. They started making it harder for Jerry and George to go places and even refused to allow George to go to Jerry's room anymore.

One time, George needed a paper signed to allow Jerry to move from one facility to another. He wasn't able to see Jerry so he gave it to Jerry's roommate, Sam, and Sam brought it to Jerry. Jerry put his "X" on it. Sam then gave it to Jerry's friend Kay, and Kay gave it back to George. When the social worker needed Jerry's verbal okay, Kay had Jerry on the pay phone and read what Jerry had told her to say.

Jerry felt as if he had fallen into a spy movie, complete with espionage, and planned to write a novel about it one day. Jerry was too short to be James Bond, so he would have to get a double, if a movie was ever made of his novel.

The night before Jerry left, every person wanted to see him to say goodbye. He was friends with all of the other people there. He would often talk with them about their concerns and worries. Kay had to make appointments for everybody to come and say goodbye. They were happy Jerry was getting out, but they were sad they wouldn't have him to talk to any longer. He was able to go back, as a visitor, several times over the years to see his old friends.

George came to see Jerry at the new facility in Torrance every month or two. George would take Jerry out for rides and talk about life. In Torrance, Jerry didn't know George would try to take out the girl in the office. George was somewhat upset when Jerry told him that he had gone out with her to her apartment. That is another story.

Years later, Jerry thought about everything that had happened during that time in his life. The only thing that really puzzled Jerry was that George would listen to Jerry but rarely shared anything about him self. George had told Jerry the barest details of what was going on in his own life. George had met and dated a lady named Lucy for months before he told Jerry anything about her. Even then, he only had mentioned her briefly in a letter. Jerry was surprised when George said he had married Lucy. Jerry didn't remember the letter right away but then it hit him that George had said something about her but it had been so off hand.

Torrance opened up a whole new world to Jerry, after George moved him there. Jerry knew the reason he was there was because George had made it happen. I was happy that Jerry realized that he needed people like George who had helped him have a better life.

At first, there was a lot more freedom at the care facility in Torrance. Jerry was able to make his own decisions about what he wanted to do. Some of the other people from the care facility, where Jerry had lived before Torrance, moved to

Torrance too. The facility in Torrance opened up a wing just for people with cerebral palsy and it was more like living in apartments than in a care facility.

But, in time, the government made the care facility follow all the rules, just like at the previous facility. Luckily, at this same time, Jerry moved to his own apartment in a complex in Orange County where eight other disabled people were moving also. This was the beginning of the In-Home Supportive Services program for seniors and disabled people. The program paid for care providers to work for people in their own homes rather than in care facilities or hospitals. This program enabled thousands of people to live independently in their own homes. Jerry never planned this but he always seemed to be in the midst of the newest thing for people with disabilities.

I knew these positive changes in Jerry's life happened because George moved Jerry out of that first care facility. If George hadn't done that, Jerry might not have been at the right place at the right time to be included in the new program. He might never have had the chance to live in his own apartment and really experience life outside of a care facility.

Section Two - Chapter 11 - Sandy, Fellow Patient

I was working on my new home that I had started after the move south. The ground, where I was digging, became hardpan at about eight inches deep so it was a hard job to dig there. I was already tired from all the moving so hitting hardpan was the last thing I needed to deal with.

Even though the rehabilitation center in Torrance, where Jerry had moved, was really just another care facility, it was a little better than the first one. Jerry seemed to be happier there and more content with his life, at least for a while. A short time after Jerry moved there he started reaching out to some of the other patients. Sandy was one of the other patients.

It started one afternoon when Jerry was pushing his chair backwards with his feet down the Fourth Wing where he lived. He knew that Sandy's room was the next room on the left. Sandy had multiple sclerosis or MS for short, unlike Jerry who had cerebral palsy. Jerry knew people with MS would eventually become worse and those like him would remain the same.

Jerry pushed his chair over to Sandy's door and sat in the doorway. Her room was all white. The aide had closed the curtains and there was a soap opera playing on the TV. There were three beds in her room but the other two patients were gone. In the bed next to the door was a tall woman with long brown hair, which flowed across the pillow. Her face was pale and clean like a child's. Her thin lips moved slightly. She said hi. Her voice was barely audible. Jerry said hello and told her his name.

The lady said, "Come in where I can see you. Sandy is my name." Jerry dug his heels into the floor and jerkily pulled his chair forward over the hump that separated the carpet in the hall and the tiles in Sandy's room. On the side of Sandy's bed was a plastic bag that caught urine from a tube coming from under Sandy's covers. Jerry wondered if that hurt her. On the nightstand, next to her bed, was a picture of a young woman that he realized was Sandy before she got so sick. There was another picture of a little boy about six. In the corner, there was a large stuffed bear. Jerry pointed at the stuffed bear and asked her who that guy in the corner was.

"That is Charley, my dancing partner," said Sandy.

He was surprised how she picked up on his speech so quickly. Not too many were able to do that. So, he asked even more questions. Jerry said that he "thought it was against the rules to dance in there."

"It is. Please don't tell." She pleaded.

Jerry said that he wouldn't if she would give him one of "those cookies on her nightstand."

"You are a black mailer." She whispered and then laughed softly.

Jerry told her he had "to eat some way." Then Jerry asked if that was a picture of her brother on the nightstand.

Sandy replied no that it was "a picture of my son Billy." And when she was well, she was going "to take care of Billy." Jerry knew people with many disabilities had sons and daughters, but Sandy was the first one he had met. Jerry had thought of becoming a father but he never had the opportunity. Looking at Sandy, Jerry doubted that she would ever be able to take care of her son but it wasn't for him to say. Jerry continued joking.

Jerry asked how she would take care of Billy if she went "dancing with Charley every night."

Sandy said that she was young enough to do both. "But, Charley was the jealous type. And that was something she would have to handle."

Jerry asked if she really "thought she could."

She replied, "No sweat."

Jerry and Sandy carried on with this light-hearted humor for months. There were times when Jerry didn't go to see Sandy. He knew Sandy was becoming worse and he didn't want to see her that way. Jerry didn't want to lose someone who he had grown to care for as a friend.

After dinner one evening, Jerry wheeled down the Fourth Wing toward his room. When he passed Sandy's room, he saw three aides working with her to tie her onto a shower chair so she wouldn't fall off. One aide closed the door as the sheet slipped off Sandy's shoulders. It was hard on Jerry to see that Sandy was getting so weak that she couldn't even sit up for a shower. Every time he saw her, she was weaker, needed more help, and gave little indication that she saw or recognized him.

After one of his last visits, Jerry slowly pushed himself down the hallway, into his room, and closed the door. He was sad and needed to be alone for a while. He realized he needed to stop going by to see her because it was so hard on her and it was just so heartbreaking for him. But he knew that he was really going to miss visiting her.

Then one day he heard that Sandy wasn't doing well and not expected to live much longer. So, after lunch, he went over to his typing table, put on his reading glasses, and pulled the string, which switched on the light over his typewriter.

Jerry typed, "Sandy, I love you."

Section Two - Chapter 12 - Bill, Physical Therapist

Gopher here again. Jerry became friends with Bill, who wasn't a physical therapist, but the care facility had hired him to work under a licensed physical therapist. The licensed therapist didn't come around much, so Bill was running the whole therapy department. Things were fairly casual, while Bill was in charge.

Jerry never was satisfied with the way things were for people with disabilities. At the same time, he wasn't one to get out and openly protest. Except for writing letters to editor of the local newspaper, he would rather just sit back and watch things unfold. For a while, he had a taste for wine. When Jerry had some wine, he didn't have any problem expressing his concepts for the future of people with disabilities.

There was the night that Bill was off duty and came to visit Jerry when Jerry was having his own party. It went something like this. Jerry had placed the water pitcher, which was full of wine, on the tray that was on wheels. He had pulled the wheeled tray around to the other side of his bed where if someone passed by his room and looked in, it would appear as if Jerry was merely drinking water. As for myself, as much as I enjoy the smell of wine, I preferred the juice from the roots of a two hundred year old walnut tree.

Suddenly, the door flew open, Jerry jumped backwards, and I hid under Jerry's bed.

"What's happening?" said Bill, as he burst into the room.

"Bill, you scared me." Jerry said.

Bill laughed. "John the janitor, and the deliverer of your wine, told me that you were having a party and I thought I would join you."

I said to myself, "Oh boy, this is going to be good. I'd better get out my lap top so I can get it all down."

Jerry said to Bill, "Sure, but close that door so nobody will see us. No one has caught me drinking in my room yet. Let's not wreck my record." Jerry had been drinking wine most nights during the entire year he had been in the facility. He didn't like being there and drank to numb himself to his surroundings. The first hospital was really awful and this one was only a slight improvement. He had tried, but he was never very happy living there.

"We must keep up your good record." Said Bill cheerfully. He quickly closed the door, came across, and sat down on Jerry's bed. "I didn't come empty handed." He pulled a bottle from under his shirt and poured some more wine into the pitcher. Then he took a drink from the bottle.

Watching Bill swig wine from the bottle, I thought, "Now, I will have to work harder to understand both of them."

Jerry took a sip from his straw. "This is good stuff."

"Yes" said Bill, as he took another gulp from the bottle of wine. "Jerry, I guess you know they are cutting back on help. Hey, I am sure you have some good ideas on how a place like this should operate. Jerry, I bet you would make a great administrator."

"Yes, I do have lots of ideas," Jerry said, "but, they are all merely part of a daydream that I have once in a while."

"Tell me more about it," Bill took another swig of wine and leaned back on one elbow.

"Well Bill, I would have a handicapped person do the interviewing of new aides and orderlies. I would want someone with a speech defect to be involved in the process too."

"Not another one I have to try to understand." I thought.

"Why do you think someone with a speech problem is needed?" Bill asked Jerry. "You know not everyone who lives here has a speech defect."

"Yes, but some do and what better way to see if someone could work with a disabled person? Speech problems are what shock new aides and orderlies right off the bat. They never have had any contact with anyone with a speech defect before."

Jerry also explained that he "would have the same morning and evening aides taking care of the same patients all the time."

"Why is that important?" said Bill, who then drained the last few drops out of his bottle of wine.

"It makes patients nervous having a different aide helping them every day. The consistency would allow the aides to know what each patient needed."

Bill thought out loud about what Jerry had said. "If patients had the same aides, I could show them what I am doing in therapy and they could follow through with it when working with the patients. I have been trying to teach a guy how to put on his own shirt but each morning an aide puts it on for him. They have no idea that I have been trying to work with the patient on that skill."

Jerry said, "That kind of thing wouldn't happen in my hospital. Each aide would check with the therapist at least once a month to see what the patient is doing in therapy. The therapist could come down on the floor any time he felt the aide needed some guidance about working with a patient such as helping the patient get dressed on their own."

"That would require that the therapists would have flexible schedules." Said Bill, warming to the subject.

"The therapist could set his own hours, as long as they added up to eight or ten hours?"

"Ten hours?"

"Yes, he would be on call twenty-four hours." Said Jerry, ignoring Bill's response, and sucking more wine up his straw.

"On call!" yelped Bill.

"That's right. But, of course, he would make forty dollars an hour, as a therapist, instead of this fifteen dollars an hour stuff."

"Now you are talking." Said Bill, warming to the subject again.

"The aides would make at least $15.00 an hour. Each aide would be required to take a special interest in at least one of the patients she has."

"You know around here aides are told not to get personally involved with any patients." Bill threw in. "In fact, if the front office knew I was talking to you like this, my job would be on the line."

"Penalizing people for reaching out and getting to know each other is unnatural. That is another thing that would have to change." Jerry said with some force. Some staff members lost their jobs, in the past, for getting too involved with Jerry. "How could an aide or therapist help any patient without taking a sincere interest in the patient?"

"They can't, but that goes for any kind of relationship. If a husband and wife don't really communicate their feelings to each other, their marriage goes on the rocks. But, Jerry, how would there be enough aides and therapists to take such an interest in each patient?"

"Oh Bill, I forgot to tell you. There will only be twenty or thirty patients in my hospital and the staff would be at least twenty. People like John, who mop the floors, would also be required to take a special interest in particular patients."

Bill took another drink. "It sounds like you have this all planned out."

"You bet I do and would you pour more wine in my glass, please." Said Jerry, barely slowing down to take a breath. "Rehabilitation for people with cerebral palsy is completely different from rehabilitation for someone who has been in a car wreck or someone who is recovering from a stroke."

"They both need to learn to walk or help themselves in some way."

"Yes, but, a person with cerebral palsy doesn't know what it is to walk like someone who has had a stroke. People recovering from an injury know what it's like to be able to walk because they had done it. Look, Bill, even though I want to walk and sometimes I daydream about it, I honestly don't know what it is like."

Bill replied "I'm beginning to see what you mean." He took another sip of wine. "For someone with cerebral palsy, it's more important to learn to use what he has. For example, you have control over your left hand and you learned to use your left hand to type with a stick."

"That's right. Using what we have instead of pushing so hard to do something that may be almost impossible to accomplish, like walking for me is."

It occurs to me, while listening to them talk about these issues, that Jerry has really put the little control he has to good use in order to have a fulfilling life. I hope he will continue to work with what he has.

After considering what Jerry was saying, Bill commented, "Maybe, I have been pushing walking too much."

"No. It's something I wanted to put all my energy into for a while. I had to know whether I ever could do it or not. I have come around to the realization that my body just cannot handle the stress and forces that trying to walk put on it. I am ready to focus my energy in different directions and pursue my writing and other interests that have been on hold."

Jerry was so adamant about his feelings on this subject that he was speaking so fast Bill couldn't keep up. Of course, the wine he was drinking wasn't helping. Sometimes Jerry had to repeat what he said because the look on Bill's face told him that Bill wasn't getting it. I needed the repeats too, as I was trying to get it all down in my computer. I could feel a book coming together just about the topic they were discussing.

"I think I agree with you about walking, at least in your case. Some people might have a different situation. Tell me more about your dream hospital."

"Each patient would have to do something with his life, such as writing, painting, volunteering, community service, etc., before I'd let him move in. And, if he reaches the point where he wasn't developing himself, he would be asked to leave."

"Wow, you would be a tough administrator." Bill had certainly never heard about any hospital like that. He leaned back on Jerry's pillows to get more comfortable.

"Give me a little more wine, please." Said Jerry, who was really getting into his subject now.

"Of course, Mr. Administrator."

"It wouldn't be called a hospital. It would be a home for active people with handicaps. The staff wouldn't call them patients. The staff would call them residents. They merely would be people or residents who need help." Jerry went on. "I would want a handicapped person, who is in a wheelchair, to help design the building. Someone in a wheelchair wouldn't put steps where a ramp should be."

"You are right about that one. Most hospitals have steps and you have to go half-way around the place to find a ramp."

"My place would be built on one level. It would have two or three small dining rooms where people could go eat instead of having one big mess hall like the army. People would have a choice of meals and those who had trouble chewing, like many with cerebral palsy, could see their food before it's ground up. Some patients here are fed meat that was pureed a week ago and some of it is warmed every evening."

Bill jumped right in, "I don't know how anyone can eat some of that stuff. There are three or four kinds of meat that are all mixed together." He made a scrunched up face of distaste, "What else would you have in your place?"

"Well, each dining room would be painted a different color and if I couldn't have but one dining room, there would be large paintings on the walls which could be changed seasonally or once every six months. Also, I would have an activity room."

"They have a craft room here and nobody likes it." Responded Bill.

"Because they are forced to make what the lady brings in and the craft hour is a part of the hospital daily routine. My activity room would have things that people living there pay for out of their own money. Also, in this room, I would have games such as chess and checkers. So, for example, if a person is learning to draw and things aren't going well he could still spend time in this room playing checkers or working on something else."

"You mean they could use this room to take their minds off problems and then go back to what they were doing?"

"Exactly! Doesn't everyone need a break once in a while?"

"I know I sure do or I would go bananas." Bill said pouring himself another glass of wine.

"People, who would be trying to overcome handicaps, may feel that way more often than other people."

"You should know."

"Another thing, I would arrange things in my place so each person living there would have a say in how his own room is fixed up. He could pay to have it painted and decorated the way he wanted. The person could make payments each month until they paid for the interior decorating like someone paying rent. That way Medicaid or the state wouldn't have to pay the entire bill for upkeep on the place." While listening to the conversation I kept wondering where the money would come from? If certain politicians get their way, it won't make any difference. People like Jerry will be living under freeway overpasses.

Jerry continued. "The main thing about this place would be every person living there would feel that it was their home. Each one would have a key to his own room, just like someone living in an apartment, so he could lock it when he left. He wouldn't have to sign in and out when he left, as patients do in the hospital." Signing in and out was one thing Jerry truly hated. He wanted the freedom to come and go whenever he pleased. He wanted his privacy. I couldn't blame him. I liked going wherever I wanted to go too.

"You would have to have some rules." Bill said.

"I would make it clear that the place was their home and they needed to make a good impression when they are out in public. I wouldn't see anything wrong, if they went to a bar and had a few drinks. If they could hold their liquor okay. In fact, they could drink in their rooms, if they wanted. So they would not have to sneak around to do it. As so many do now. But if someone drinks all the time and doesn't try to improve them self in some way, they would be asked to leave."

I'm thinking that Jerry acts as if he is already there in the new place.

"That's true in any situation." Said Bill taking another sip of his wine, "Everybody needs some freedom and to be responsible for themselves."

"That is exactly what I'm talking about." Jerry said rather excitedly.

"Have you thought about having married people in your place?"

"Yes, people with disabilities need and want relationships. Just like everyone else. Being with someone is very important. It is the biggest frustration for people living in institutions."

"Then, how would you handle it?" Bill asked, thinking that since Jerry had ideas about everything else, he would have some insight into this issue too.

"Well, what people do in their own rooms would be their own business. I surely wouldn't try to hide sex from handicapped people like most hospitals do. Acting as though sexual desires don't exist for a disabled person causes them to feel odd and be depressed and confused."

"What if an aide becomes very involved with a patient and spends three nights in his room?"

"First, if the aide kept doing her work and the patient continued to show he was developing himself in what ever he was doing, I wouldn't say anything."

"You really know what you are talking about."

"After all, I have been in a care facility setting my whole adult life."

Bill finished the wine. "When you open your place, will you give me a job?"

"I will think about it."

A few months later, Jerry moved out of that place and began experiencing life on the outside. Come on and I will tell you what happened.

Section Three
Chapters 13 thru 21

Jerry, Age 30-50
Independent Living

Section Three - Chapter 13 - Brad, Jerry's Care Provider

When Jerry was living in southern California, he went through a great number of care providers. Brad was one of the best and they both could look back on the time they spent together and smile. From a gopher's point of view, some of the things that happened were questionable.

Brad was also a care provider for another gentleman with cerebral palsy. His name was Sidney. Sidney was very hard on Brad. One time, Brad came over to Jerry's and Brad looked like he had been in a fight. His eyes and his whole body looked like somebody had been punching him. Jerry asked what was going on. Brad didn't want to talk about it. About three months later, Brad decided not to work for Sidney any longer. A girl, named Megan, worked for Sidney after that. Brad had an easier time helping Jerry after he stopped working for Sidney.

One day, Brad decided he would make a dinner of homemade enchiladas for Jerry. This was because for some time Jerry had been giving Brad a bad time about not being able to cook.

The day came to make the enchiladas and Brad worked a long time on them. That afternoon, Brad came back from helping somebody else and went into the kitchen to get the enchiladas ready for Jerry's dinner.

Brad put the enchiladas on a plate and cut them into small pieces so Jerry wouldn't choke on them.

Right before he was going to give Jerry a bite, Brad said wait a minute; he had forgotten something. He reached into the icebox and before Jerry had known what was going on Brad put barbeque sauce on the enchiladas.

Jerry and Brad looked at each other. Jerry asked Brad if he knew what he had done. Brad said yep, he knew what he had done; he had put barbeque sauce on the enchiladas. Jerry just looked at him and nodded. Brad then realized he had meant to grab the taco sauce and not the barbeque sauce.

Brad was very upset and called himself all kinds of names. Jerry said every body makes mistakes; but he had never anticipated this one.

Brad got up and tried to take the barbeque sauce off the enchiladas, but it was impossible. So, the next thing he tried was to get the extra enchiladas from the freezer and defrost them. Jerry realized that they had only been in the freezer for half an hour and would defrost quickly. A little while later, they had a nice dinner of enchiladas.

Brad helped Jerry with many things. At times, it looked like a comedy of errors. One time, a radio station was going to interview Jerry on the radio about having started the first dating service for people with disabilities. This dating service was a place to introduce disabled people to each other.

Jerry had written out something he wanted to have Brad say for him during the interview. Brad was going to read Jerry's comments during the interview on the phone from Brad's apartment. One problem, Brad forgot to take home the comments that Jerry had written. So, Brad had to wing it. He did a good job, but Jerry was at home holding his breath and hoping Brad wouldn't promise something that Jerry couldn't do.

Brad never knew what Jerry might need or want him to do. Once, Brad walked into Jerry's apartment and Jerry was holding a broken part from his wheelchair. Jerry said they were going across town to get this thing fixed. Brad said okay without much enthusiasm. Then he helped Jerry into the car and they drove half way across town to a place that fixed the wheelchair part.

Sometimes Brad and Jerry went out to eat at a restaurant called Marie Calendar's. Brad always ordered a quiche. He told Jerry not to get the wrong idea, that he, Brad, was not a wimp because he ate quiche. This had taken place in the early 1980's at a time when it wasn't considered manly to eat quiche. Jerry ate quiche too, but he had to eat soft food, so he had an excuse! I knew I was just a mere gopher, but I tried quiche and I liked it. What's the problem with quiche? These guys were crazy to worry about what they ate. But who am I to say? I just dig tunnels.

Brad helped Jerry to realize that Jerry needed help to wash his privates because he wasn't getting clean by doing it himself. This was very hard for Jerry. When the new aide was hired, Brad told the aide how to wash Jerry correctly.

I was able to understand how Jerry would feel awkward and this was the beginning of giving up some independence. That was very hard for him to do, as keeping his independence was very important to him.

Section Three - Chapter 14 - Michael, Pam's Son

For a while, Jerry had a neighbor, Pam, who worked for him as a caregiver and she had a little boy named Michael. Michael decided that Jerry was someone that he liked. Michael was about two when he met Jerry.

Jerry had always wanted to be a father and he would have been a good one. So Michael coming into his life was one of the best things that could have happened.   He had all the abilities to father a child but he never got to do that partly because he was so wrapped up in his writing and partly because he never met the "right" woman. But Michael came into Jerry's life and kind of satisfied this longing in Jerry.

 When Michael's mother came to work, he would come with her. He would get on the table and watch when his mother fed Jerry. One day, his mom walked away for a minute and Michael picked up the spoon and started feeding Jerry. When Michael thought about it for a minute, he ended up taking a bite after Jerry. Then it was one bite for Jerry and one bite for him. This was how they did it from then on.

Jerry could take his pills on his own, if they were stuck in marshmallows and placed on a mat. The mat was on a rolling typing table. Jerry moved that typing table wherever he needed it. Sometimes it was by his computer or near his bed.

One time, when Jerry and Michael's mom turned around, they saw that all the marshmallows on the table were gone. Jerry and Michael's mom started thinking that maybe they should call an ambulance. They were afraid of what the pills would do to Michael. But when they took a better look, they realized Michael had removed all of the pills and just eaten the marshmallows. Michael had then carefully placed the pills back on the table exactly where they had been but without the marshmallows under them. Whew, what a relief they both felt. Jerry decided to take advantage of Michael's intelligence. He

wasn't aware at that point of just how cunning and crafty
Michael would grow to be.

When Jerry needed his safety belt buckled on his electric
chair, Michael would stand on Jerry's footrests and buckle it
for him. When Jerry went for his mail, Michael would crawl
up on Jerry's lap and ride to the mailbox. Then Michael would
get down and get Jerry's mail for him. Then Michael would
show Jerry each one and Jerry would tell him keep it or throw
it away. This became a daily occurrence for them both.
Michael would see the mailman come and rush to Jerry's
apartment and get Jerry into his power chair and they would go
check the mail.

One day, Michael's dad had to work, and was unable to go
to see Michael's play at school. So Jerry showed up to watch
the play and when Michael saw Jerry he smiled. His friend
was there to show support. Jerry felt just like a proud father
that day.

When Jerry would return from the store, Michael would
put the groceries away for Jerry. Then, one day, Michael
asked Jerry if people were paid for helping him and Jerry said
yes. After that, Michael asked for a quarter for the job of
putting away Jerry's groceries. Jerry knew then that Michael
would be a good businessman. Also, Michael reminded Jerry
of himself when he was kid and had asked his dad for a quarter
for mopping the floor.

There was that night when Michael asked Jerry two
questions and Jerry wasn't sure he had good answers for him.
Michael asked if Jerry believed in God. Jerry replied yes.
Then Michael asked him, if he believed in God, why he didn't
ask God to heal him from having disabilities. Jerry replied that
God used him with his disabilities to help other people. That
answer satisfied Michael. But, years later, Jerry wanted to add
that having disabilities had given Jerry the chance to
experience being a father to Michael.

Another day, Jerry needed to have someone change a wheel on his wheelchair. Michael's dad told Michael to go work on it and when Michael was done his dad would check it to make sure everything was okay. Michael worked so long that Michael's mother had to come over and get Michael because he had fallen asleep on Jerry's feet.

Michael said he wanted to join the Air Force and fly planes when he was older. He was even interested in becoming an astronaut. Jerry never has heard from Michael since moving from southern California. There are times when Jerry hears about a plane going down in enemy territory. Jerry always says a silent prayer that it isn't his Michael.

Section Three - Chapter 15 - David, Wheelchair Guy

Those, who know Jerry now, think of him as driving a power chair all over town to stores and coffee cafés. This was not always the case. For a long time, Jerry got places by pushing himself backwards in his manual wheelchair. Early in the 1980's, David was the one who got Jerry his first durable and fully-usable power wheelchair.

Jerry received his first power wheelchair specifically to get him around Long Beach State University. That first power chair did not have any electric brakes. Jerry needed to pull back on the joystick to make it stop. He kept it at the college and used it there exclusively for about a year.

Then Jerry brought it home and used it to go to the store. The makers of this wheelchair didn't build it to go to the store or anywhere else. It was dangerous. But Jerry needed the freedom to go anywhere he wanted to go.

It was about that time that Jerry met David. David was new to working on power wheelchairs. As new as he was to working on power wheelchairs, David still knew right away that Jerry needed a new chair. This is how the whole thing got started. David wanted to give Jerry more freedom. As a gopher, who had watched Jerry for a while, I wondered if Jerry was ready for more freedom. And, too, was the world prepared for Jerry. He had been living on his own for just two and a half years. Jerry still had a lot to learn about life. Being in care facilities for some time, Jerry figured that he was behind about ten years in learning things. Jerry wanted to make up for lost time.

David first ordered a wheelchair that the manufacture hadn't made to take the abuse that Jerry would give it. Jerry broke the front wheel forks on the chair about every two weeks, when he went up and down driveways and the cuts in the curbs. These curb cuts were not even with the street surface and this put a lot of force on the structure of the chair.

After a while, Jerry figured out if he went at an angle, he was able to go up and down curb cuts without putting so much force on the chair. This gave him more time with the wheel forks before they broke. This made David happy for a while. John, Jerry's friend, would keep extra wheelchair forks and tools in his car. In case Jerry broke down, no matter where that might be, John was prepared to repair the wheelchair.

Then, about three years later, David ordered a new chair with heavy-duty forks. They thought, no problem; but actually, their problems had just begun. The problem with Jerry's newest chair was the joystick. It would not hold up to the abuse that Jerry's hand would put it through. Jerry had a lot of strength in his left hand but little control over how hard he pushed the joystick.

The electrical parts that controlled the joystick weren't well constructed or reliable. One time, the joystick control went crazy and Jerry went around and around in circles. It would also go into high gear while going around in circles and Jerry called David to get over there as Jerry was getting dizzy.

David called the company, which was back east, that made the joystick and they told him to mail it to them. David got the joystick back to the company that designed it and they had it for over a week. But, when the wheelchair company returned the joystick, it still didn't function correctly. David was getting angry at the whole situation.

Also, David was scared that the chair would again start going around and around in circles with Jerry trapped in it. The next time, Jerry really could get hurt. David called the company and asked them to send the instructions on setting the controls for the joystick and they told him they couldn't give him that information.

David decided that this was the last go around with that company.   David opened the box and tried fixing it himself. Jerry was right there at the table to watch. David thought that the wires were going to be different colors and he could easily trace which wires led to the controller that made the chair go forward and back and which ones made the chair move right and left. He also thought he could easily isolate the wire for controlling the speed too.

But when David opened the joystick controller box, the wires were only black and white. David had to test each wire to see where it led. After almost three hours, David got the controller box back together and the chair ran great.

The next Christmas, Jerry had a shirt made for David that said Wheelchair King.

Section Three - Chapter 16 - Sally, Haircut Lady

Now, being a gopher, I was able to see things about Jerry that most people could never imagine. Things like the subject of sex, which didn't come up often when it came to persons with disabilities. But, either Jerry forgot that he was disabled or people didn't know how able he was in this aspect of life. I knew Jerry was not a stranger to that need and he went to great trouble to fulfill this desire. I hope I don't get too embarrassed telling you.

For a while, Jerry would visit bars. He did this partly because he had a job at a center for the disabled where he was given assignments impossible for anyone to do and partly just to prove he could. If, something seemed impossible for him to do, he would try it just to say he had tried it.

Anyway, Jerry met a nice lady named Sally in a bar. For a while, they just talked about things such as Jerry being a writer and that she had two daughters and a son. Each evening would end with Jerry inviting Sally over to his apartment and she declining saying something like, "I've got to get home," as if she had to get home because she had an early morning. They would kiss and Jerry would make it home in his power chair. Each time Jerry would ask her to come over; she kept making excuses for not coming home with him.

Then, one night Jerry didn't have any alcohol to drink because he was planning to finish a report for the center. As usual, Jerry asked Sally about coming home with him. When Sally said "yes," Jerry was at a loss for words. Sally followed in her car as Jerry drove his power chair home.

In time, Jerry relaxed. Sally and Jerry spent a beautiful evening together. "That was the nicest evening I have had in a long time." Sally told him

Jerry replied, "It was the same for me."

After such a beautiful night, Jerry started calling Sally and asking her to come over. It turned out that Sally happened to be a barber. This was the perfect excuse, if anyone asked Jerry why the woman was coming to his apartment. He could just say he needed a haircut. Sally couldn't understand Jerry's speech very well so she would ask if he needed a haircut. If Jerry said, "yes," Sally knew it was going to be a romantic evening and explained she had to go by her home first to check on her daughter. She then would ask if nine o'clock was okay. Jerry would tell her that was all right.

Then Jerry would hurry up and call his care provider to tell her that she didn't have to come back that evening to put him to bed. This became a regular thing. They both enjoyed those evenings together. Sometimes, two or three months would go by when they didn't see each other, yet, whenever one called the other, they got together.

After about two years, Jerry met someone else who fit better into other areas of his life. Sally and Jerry went their separate ways. They still spoke on the phone occasionally. Sometimes, they both thought back about the nice evenings they had spent together. He ran into her later on and she told him that she had gotten a part-time job at a convalescent hospital. Perhaps, knowing Jerry helped her to be a good care provider. They had developed a special friendship with each other.

Section Three - Chapter 17 - Dorothy, Jerry's Girlfriend

Dorothy was with Jerry when he experienced both great joy and deep sadness. Jerry had stopped working as a writer at the independent living center and had started a dating service for people with disabilities. This was before he had a computer so he had to use his electric typewriter to do all the correspondence for his business. The local newspaper had done a piece about his business. So he had many people contacting him and was very busy dealing with the success of his business.

Dorothy had read the article and offered to help with the paper work in exchange for a free membership. The truth was that Dorothy was interested in Jerry. It took Jerry quite a while to realize why Dorothy was coming over at times when there wasn't any work for her to do. Dorothy thought Jerry wasn't interested and almost gave up on the guy.

But, after Jerry finally made a move, Dorothy and Jerry had a beautiful relationship for several years. They went out to eat, to Disneyland, to the movies, to concerts, and traveled up and down California. Jerry kind of blew going out to the movies when he showed her how to work a VCR. After that, every Friday evening, Dorothy would show up with food for three days and six or seven movies. Sometimes they didn't even bother getting dressed.

One night, when they were on their way out to dinner, they had to stop by his mother's to loan her some money. Just before Jerry's mom got to the car, Dorothy put money from her purse into Jerry's hand for him to give to his mom. This was so that Jerry could be the one giving his mom money and not Dorothy.

Jerry thought they had a future together. But, in the back of his mind, Jerry thought Dorothy was keeping something from him. Jerry didn't know exactly how to ask her. Jerry thought Dorothy certainly had the right to keep some things in the past to herself. Her son let the cat out of the bag one morning at breakfast, when Jerry and Dorothy were visiting her son and his family in San Jose.

Her son casually mentioned the mobile home Dorothy was planning on buying and asked how Jerry would get into it in his wheelchair. He mentioned building a ramp, but it was obvious that Dorothy wasn't planning on taking Jerry or building a ramp into the mobile home for him. Jerry had no idea she was planning to move or to buy a mobile home. Everyone at the table got very quiet and one by one, they got up and left the table.

On the way home from that trip, Jerry cried most of the way and Dorothy was very quiet. Dorothy certainly didn't want to hurt Jerry that way. But shortly after that, they decided to break up. Jerry cried for two weeks after Dorothy left and he wasn't able to listen to anything on the radio that reminded him of Dorothy.

It wasn't too long after Dorothy and Jerry had broken up that Jerry received word that his mom had had a stroke and was in the hospital. One of Jerry's neighbors told Jerry to call Dorothy. Jerry was reluctant for a while but he finally called Dorothy. Dorothy came as soon as she could.

Dorothy stayed with Jerry at the hospital as much as possible. Besides dealing with his mom's situation, Jerry also had to contend with Lance and their Aunt Ruth, who both tended to twist things around. Dorothy would hold him every night. She would explain what had really happened that day at the hospital. Lance and their Aunt Ruth were continuously confusing him by telling him different things.

When Jerry was visiting his mom for many hours every day, Dorothy would bring him something to eat at the hospital. This was because the hospital cafeteria didn't have anything he could eat. His brother and aunt were too upset about his mom dying to think about the idea that he might be hungry.

It was very hard on Jerry during his mom's hospital stay and after her death. It was made even more difficult because Lance and Aunt Ruth blamed him for agreeing to the surgeries that the doctors did. He really needed Dorothy in his life right then to help him get through it all.

After Jerry's mom passed away, Dorothy stayed around for almost a year. He and Dorothy went back to their old routine. Dorothy made him feel like a real person in many ways. Dorothy asked him for his opinion about problems at home and at work. But Dorothy never discussed her moving away with Jerry. Eventually, she just told him she was going to move and she did. She moved north as she had planned to do before his mother died. He wasn't upset because he had already gone through it one time before.

Dorothy was very special to Jerry and he never understood how she just moved away and never contacted him again except for one visit she made with her new roommate. Jerry always wondered if Dorothy would have stayed, if he had given up drinking.

I knew some things in life were hard and I was sad for Jerry when Dorothy left. I knew Jerry might never completely get over Dorothy's leaving. He had other relationships with women but none like the one he had had with Dorothy. He had called her his girlfriend and she was the one complete relationship in his life.

Before meeting Dorothy, Jerry wasn't sure he would ever have a close and rewarding relationship with a woman. Afterwards, Jerry knew he could have as normal a relationship with the right woman as any man.

Section Three - Chapter 18 - Long Beach State University

Jerry got into many odd situations while he was attending Long Beach State University. Right off the bat, Jerry went against the normal way of doing things. As you read this book, you will learn Jerry didn't do many things like other people. Being someone with disabilities truly didn't influence this trait in Jerry. He was born to be a little different. The world was Jerry's test track. Like a racecar driver, Jerry had to find out just how far he could take something.

After taking only two writing courses at a junior college, a teacher encouraged Jerry to go on to a university. Since Jerry was only planning to take writing classes, he had to find a way to pass the entrance examination. Jerry used common sense for the science part. For history, Jerry remembered enough from high school to get through. But math was a problem. A friend told Jerry just to answer each math problem by checking the second answer for every question. Jerry did this. The guy who was writing down the answers gave Jerry a questioning look. Jerry got a high score in English and grammar. That was not a surprise to anybody. He also passed the math section.

Jerry's first class at the university was very hard and frustrating because the teacher wouldn't call on him and told him to put his hand down every time he raised it. That was very different from the community college teacher who made sure he had a chance to take an active part in the class. Since Jerry needed this first class to advance to higher writing classes, he didn't make a big deal. He just did what the teacher wanted and handed in the assignments.

Meanwhile, Jerry made friends with the man who was the head of the creative writing department and he told Jerry what class to take next time. The second class at the university was very satisfying for Jerry.

After Jerry had been at the university two or three years, he thought he was a hotshot writer. Some teachers encouraged him to take a class from Dr. Smith. After reading Jerry's best story, Mr. Smith said that Jerry did not know much about writing. But, if Jerry would work, Mr. Smith would try to improve Jerry's writing. Jerry worked with Mr. Smith about three years. Mr. Smith then stated Jerry's writing was somewhat better.

While Jerry was working with Mr. Smith on a novel, he also became the editor of the university's newsletter for people with disabilities. Jerry became quite good at balancing two or more activities at once. Jerry is still doing that balancing thing, but now being over sixty, he reluctantly admits he can't keep track of as many projects as he once did. And it doesn't matter how many more hard drives and thumb drives he adds to his computer. His own memory is just not there.

When Jerry had first started attending Long Beach State University, the disability department had to share a phone with the religious studies department. Jerry never really figured out why these two departments had the same phone number except they both gave out help. I thought, if the disability department couldn't help someone, it would be easy just to slip them to the religious studies department by pushing one button. That saved on the paper work I guess. Like Jerry, I learned when not to ask too many questions. Some people get nervous with questions.

During Jerry's years at the university, the department for students with disabilities had two directors named David. The first David had had polio as a child and only had use of one hand. This was before there were any laws stating schools had to provide special help to people like Jerry who couldn't feed themselves. So the first David would use his good hand to feed lunch to Jerry. Before the first David was director of disabled student services he had worked where people came and played games. His job had been to give a number to people who had wanted to play pool. He told Jerry that feeding him was like shooting a ball in the corner pocket. When this first David died, Jerry wrote a humorous piece for the service that they held at the university for David. But they didn't read it at the service. He really was never sure why they didn't. Maybe they didn't appreciate the humorous, inside jokes he included. He always thought David would have gotten the jokes, but maybe nobody else did.

The second David came on board about a month later. When Jerry met him, this David had long hair and he did not look like the director of a department. When other people met him, they had their doubts too. But, before it was over, he was able to get almost the whole floor for the disabled students department. The second David also set up a program that paid other students to feed Jerry.

When the state rehabilitation department didn't want to pay Jerry's way through school any longer, the second David went with Jerry to the hearing. The people from rehab had a whole table of files about his case at the hearing. David just had one card with a few notes on it. David made them realize that Jerry truly belonged in school and the department of rehabilitation granted him two additional years at the university.

Section Three - Chapter 19 - Another Job

Jerry didn't get enough work at the disabled students department at Long Beach State University, so he turned around and went to work for an agency that helped disabled people be as independent as possible. It also hired disabled people to do the work. He had thought, oh boy, just what he needed.

Jerry was happy at first, but soon he was just disappointed. I had been around Jerry long enough to know he wasn't going to be happy there. He wanted things to be done right and most agencies would cut corners and didn't do what they set out to do.

A government grant funded Jerry's job. Under the program, he would work from four to eighteen months. Then, after that, the agency had the choice to hire him as part of the regular staff or not. His job was to look at the new laws passed by the legislature that pertained to the disabled. And then he would re-write them in language that people were able to understand.

Jerry got his hopes up because it seemed that he was doing his duties well. But soon he realized the reason he got the job was that he had the most obvious physical handicaps for government people to see when they came to observe the program. Most other workers were blind or hard of hearing. Their disabilities didn't have the visual impact of someone like Jerry who was in a wheelchair.

But, Jerry met many new people at the agency. Like the woman who worked with the deaf people. One day, a man asked the woman what Jerry had just said. The woman then mimicked Jerry's speech and sounded just like him. It was funny the way that man just walked away looking very confused.

Another lady, Nancy, that Jerry met at the agency, was blind or going blind at the time. Everybody who worked there told Jerry not to stop or wait in the hallway. But once, Jerry was just in the hallway for a few minutes waiting to see someone. The receptionist told Nancy she had a phone call. Nancy said she would take the call in her office and she went down the hallway and ran right into Jerry and his wheelchair. After that, Jerry always wore aftershave so she could smell him and know he was there.

Remember, Jerry did not have a computer in those days, nearly 25 years ago. So whatever he did, he did one letter at a time with a stick on an electric typewriter. Using the typewriter was causing problems with his arm. His arm was going numb sometimes and he had to pick it up with his other arm and put it on the keyboard.

One time, the woman who put out the newsletter was sick and Jerry thought this was his time to prove what he could do. He had done many newsletter layouts at his other job at Long Beach State University. He went to the conference room and he and his helper laid out the pages by hand. He used white sheets of paper and numbered them all. He then put stories on each one of the pieces of paper and he made sure they went the right way.

After doing the newsletter layout, Jerry thought they didn't recognize him for what he could do. He just needed a thank you or someone there to say that he did a good job. This never happened.

At one point, Jerry tried for two weeks to get the executive director, Margaret, to look at what he had done. But she always was too busy or she would tell him she was going to do it later the next day. Her behavior towards him made him feel unimportant. He also wondered if he should remain there when the woman obviously did not respect him or what he was doing.

About three months before the grant that covered Jerry's job at the agency was going to end, the blind woman, Nancy, became his supervisor. They both wondered how this was going to work. Nancy wasn't able to see Jerry's letter board or read a note that he typed. They both decided that somehow they would make it work anyway.

Nancy was able to hear better than most, possibly because she was blind. So she got Jerry to speak slower so she was able to understand him. When she realized how much Jerry was able to do, she was amazed but she still didn't know where they were able to use him. Soon they became good friends.

Jerry was almost a real employee. Each employee was required to answer the phone for an hour a week. They thought okay, they could put him on the phones on Friday from three to four with a lady who understood his speech. Nobody important will call on Friday. He felt important though.

But, Jerry made a mistake. Somebody who needed a place to sleep that night, called the center. Jerry approved the money for the room and twenty dollars more for meals. Jerry was happy that he could help someone. Monday morning, when Margaret, the director, looked at the log she almost had a heart attack. She came to Jerry and asked him if he knew that he needed to get approval for a room and meals. Jerry told her yes but he was the only one there besides the girl who helped him on the phone. And besides, he proudly said, that he was the "officer of the day."

The next week, Jerry's shift was for only a half an hour, starting at four thirty in the afternoon. Since the agency closed at five o'clock, they hoped Jerry would not have enough time to make any more mistakes.

Once, they hired a guy who worked with Jerry on the newsletter. They both had one major article to write and the articles were due in six weeks. Jerry did his piece in about a week and put it in his briefcase.

The other guy asked Jerry about three times what to do about the article he was supposed to write. Jerry told him to go to the deaf students department and interview one of the people there. Jerry didn't worry about him any more. But about two days before the pieces were due, the editor asked for their articles. Jerry reached into his briefcase and pulled out his.

Then the editor asked the other guy for his and he didn't have it. The editor was very upset and asked Jerry if he would do it. So, Jerry outlined his subject, went to the woman who worked in the deaf department, and interviewed her. Then he went home and typed all night long to finish the story. He took the story to the editor the next day.

The editor did say thank you to him but she didn't include the second article he wrote in the newsletter. That didn't bother him as much as the fact that he didn't get any recognition or acknowledgement for coming through or being a good employee.

There were some weeks when Jerry didn't work. It wasn't because he was mad. They just didn't have any work for him to do. Every day around ten, Jerry would call and ask if they had anything for him to do.

One day, another guy with a similar speech problem called at the same time that Jerry usually did. The woman, who had mimicked his speech, thought it was Jerry and kidded him by saying that he needed to take the marshmallows out of his mouth as it may help him talk better. After that, the lady made sure it was Jerry before joking around on the phone.

About a year later, Nancy called Jerry and said that they had received money for five computers and told Jerry that she had arranged for him to receive one of them. This was because he would be the one that would probably use it the most. Learning to use a computer helped Jerry to go on to be a successful writer.

After Jerry had left the center, Nancy retired and they had a party for her. They invited Jerry to it and it was very nice. They had a dance and when they started playing the music, Nancy's husband went over, grabbed her hand, and took her to the dance floor. The song playing was, "You are the Wind Beneath My Wings." Jerry was so happy to have known Nancy. Even today, he cries when he hears that song.

Section Three - Chapter 20 - Violet
Afternoon Joke Teller

Violet was Jerry's afternoon care provider for at least five years. She acquired this job when his then current provider just left Jerry and Violet, the guy's girlfriend, alone in a restaurant and Jerry's dinner was sitting in front of him. Obviously, the guy who abandoned Jerry when he was supposed to be there to help wasn't a very good care provider. He had a lot of problems and was flaky to boot. But, Violet started feeding Jerry and ended up with the job on a regular basis from then on. The flaky guy was history.

Violet and Jerry had many conversations about this human being and they never figured out if this guy was good for anything. And Jerry never could figure out why Violet dated him. If Violet hadn't been dating this other guy, Jerry might have gotten romantically involved with her.

After Violet became Jerry's regular care provider, she showed up every afternoon. Jerry thought she was there to feed him but he soon realized she came to tell him jokes. So, Violet treated Jerry to a steady stream of jokes along with good cooking. Some of her jokes were quite long. So sometimes, his dinner was an hour late. Perhaps, this was good because Jerry could have choked from laughing.

Violet liked to joke about bodily functions. So, at times Jerry thought he was in junior high school. Jerry never went to junior high so Violet gave him a taste of how silly junior high school could have been. Jerry didn't think he missed much!

Soon, Jerry felt like he knew her family from the stories Violet told. Jerry could tell that her dad was quite a character. Her dad had strong opinions about world events and he drew cartoons illustrating what he felt. Most of the time, his cartoons didn't show lawmakers at their best. But at Christmas time, he would lighten up and do some joyful drawings about the season.

Her dad always made sure that Violet brought his newest creations for Jerry to see. I was always anxious and excited to see her dad's next drawing. Wasn't there a gopher way back who was an artist? I need to look that up on the Internet. Anyway, Jerry's apartment was a gallery for her dad's work.

Violet was frustrated because she was living at home with her parents. Her mom was responsible for much of Violet's frustration. Her mom loved to get and keep junk mail, daily newspapers, and many magazines. Her mom would pile all these valuables around her chair so they would be in easy reach. If Violet tried to clean up, her mom would yell that Violet was intruding on her privacy.

Once, Violet thought she could throw away some of her mom's six-month-old junk mail. She didn't think her mother would notice. But, her mother caught her. Her life was in danger until she retrieved the valuables from the trash. Violet would say, "There was stuff on the right of mom's chair, stuff on the left, and stuff in front of her chair." Jerry could relate because his mom did the same thing.

I wondered if I could have used any of that stuff to brace my tunnels. Then, I remembered junk mail was made of paper. That wouldn't have held up long.

Once, I had an emergency cave in and I thought about using some old stories Jerry had written. But, with my luck, he would have wanted to enter them into his computer right then. Believe me; he remembered everything he had ever written. There was the time he had Violet looking through his whole apartment for a story he had written ten or more years earlier. Then he decided he didn't really need that story after all. If he could have read Violet's mind, he would have run for his life. I was hiding deep down in my tunnel.

Violet's brother usually worked nights and one night he didn't have to work. He was sitting in the kitchen holding a flashlight in his mouth to read the paper because he didn't want to wake up anyone in the house. Violet walked into the kitchen to get a snack, was scared speechless, and almost did something in her nightgown. The next day, Jerry got a detailed description about this incident. His dinner was half an hour late that evening, as Violet's story about her brother was exceptionally long.

When Violet was caring for Jerry, other care providers would take advantage of him by borrowing money and never paying it back. Violet had quite a large bosom. So when Jerry wanted to get money out of his house without anyone else knowing, Violet tucked money in her bra and walked past whoever was in his apartment and went home. Violet looked so innocent. She was a church-going person! There was one bothersome thing about this arrangement. She would hand his money to him when Jerry asked. Jerry wanted to make his own withdrawals.

Because of having cerebral palsy, Jerry had a pronounced startle reflex. Every afternoon, when Violet came, she would work in the kitchen and Jerry would be working on his computer in the bedroom. She sometimes thought Jerry had heard her come in but Jerry was concentrating on learning his new computer and didn't hear anything. So when she walked into the bedroom, Jerry would jump and yell "Violet!" and throw his hands up.

Violet and Jerry cried and laughed together and they both learned about life.

Section Three - Chapter 21 - Mike, Jerry's Friend

After I was around Jerry awhile, I realized he met some interesting and maybe even odd people. Among the most unusual was Mike.

Jerry met Mike when he was going to a store where he might be able to buy a lock box. Jerry could not do fine motor movements. So, he was hoping to find a lock box that he could use on his own. Mike was the manager of the store. So, Mike searched through catalogs trying to find one that looked like it would work for Jerry.

Their new friendship seemed innocent enough, at the time, but seeing these two together made you shake your head. Mike was very friendly and Jerry stopped by to visit him frequently after that. Mike stood out in a crowd. He was six feet four inches tall and a big guy. He wore a cowboy hat and cowboy boots. He was proud of his boots.

At some point, Jerry invited Mike to his apartment. Jerry thought Mike could get a better idea of what Jerry needed. This seemed like a good idea until Mike brought wine coolers. Then, it was hard to understand anything.

One time, Mike hung Jerry's phone on the wall so Jerry could answer it. Jerry made Mike sit on the bed to get him to realize there was no possible way to reach the phone while sitting down. Mike put the phone back where Jerry had it while complaining that some people just didn't appreciate help.

Jerry knew Mike for twenty years. They were good friends all those years.

Section Four
Chapters 22 thru 28

Jerry, Age 50-67
Central California

Section Four - Chapter 22 - Betty
Jerry's Friend, Care Provider, and Editor

I remember that Jerry was still learning how to use his computer when he first emailed Betty. Emails opened up a completely new method of communicating for Jerry. Betty was about to quit getting email at home because it was just so primitive and slow back then. But then she got this email from Jerry about wanting a friend and it was interesting to her so she decided not to let her email service expire. They both didn't know they would become lifelong friends.

After a month of email back and forth and speaking to Jerry on the phone, Betty decided to go and meet the man that was doing this. It just happened to be Jerry. Betty thought to herself, as she walked towards his apartment, if this guy isn't a disabled person when I meet him, he will be afterwards. Some men wrote emails making up stories just to meet women. Betty didn't want anything like that. Luckily, for Jerry, he actually had cerebral palsy.

The first time Betty met Jerry, he was wearing red sweat pants and a red sweatshirt that had stains all over them. Jerry had bought them to go to bed in. He didn't like red but he thought they were all right for bed. Betty, the next time she came over to see him, brought him a white shirt with a red car on it. Jerry said thank you but he really hated red.

The first time Jerry went out with Betty he was watching the riots in Los Angeles on TV. Jerry didn't realize how bad they were and Betty didn't know about them at all, so he and Betty went out. Jerry wanted it to be an easy trip the first time they went somewhere. So they went to see the Dancing Waters at the Disneyland Hotel. But Jerry forgot that they had two steps to climb to get a good view. Jerry had to walk up the steps while holding on to the rail while Betty held him up and then she pulled his chair up. That wasn't the best way for

Jerry to make a good first impression. Luckily, Betty gave him another chance.

The next time they went out, Betty asked Jerry if he wanted an ice cream. He said yes. They were in a drive thru. Betty handed Jerry the cardboard carrier with the ice cream Sundays in it and they started to drive away. Then Betty noticed the nuts on top of the Sundays and realized that Jerry couldn't eat nuts. So Betty made a quick u-turn at the next street and the cups of ice cream went all over the place. Before that, Betty hadn't seen any reason why Jerry couldn't hold the carrier with the ice cream in it. She was learning just how Jerry's cerebral palsy affected what he could and couldn't do. Jerry knew right then that he would get no breaks from her about his disabilities. That was how he liked it.

In time, Jerry's life started to go down hill because of the people he had working for him. Jerry couldn't find anyone good to take care of him. Also, people he had known at various agencies were no longer at those agencies. The new people at the agencies seemed not to have time for Jerry. At one point, Jerry knew many people including neighbors, social workers, and former care providers he could call for advice and help. But things just changed before Jerry knew it. Betty did what she could and tried to keep his apartment up for him on the weekends when she wasn't working at her regular job.

Betty had a very demanding job and she was getting carpal tunnel syndrome in her hands so her job was getting difficult to continue doing and the whole situation rather unpleasant. People, where she worked, would not even try to help make it workable for her by changing her position or duties. She eventually quit her job and moved 200 miles north to another city.

At the same time, as Betty was moving north, Jerry had learned they were going to take his apartment away. They were then going to tell him where he had to live. Jerry didn't like that idea. So when Betty made an offer to Jerry to come and live with her, he was ready.

So began another time in Jerry's life and mine. Jerry got a hold of one of his old friends, George, and asked George to help him move one more time. The day Jerry was going to move, most of his caregivers came over and helped him. That night Jerry was so tired that he just lay down on a blanket on the floor after everybody had packed the truck. He just laid there with his head on the floor, resting, and covering his eyes with the hat that Betty had bought him on a trip they had taken to San Diego. One of his former caregivers, who had come over to help him move, was just leaning back against the wall until it was time to get Jerry ready. Then she got him up and fed him some food. She told him goodbye with tears in her eyes.

Jerry's friend George and all of Jerry's belongings took off to the Central Valley to Betty's house. Jerry was so tired that he ended up sleeping seat belted in, so he wouldn't fall over, all the way to the Central Valley. I went too, of course, and it was a hard ride on that U-Haul bumper. But I wanted to know what new adventures were in store for Jerry.

When we arrived at Betty's home, she was not there, so George began unloading Jerry's stuff in the front yard. Betty had gone to the market to buy groceries so she wouldn't have to go after Jerry got there. She hadn't expected them to arrive quite so early. When Betty came back, she asked George to put Jerry's furniture in the house. George ate a whole bag of chips that Betty had just bought, while he was in there, as he was so hungry.

It took a little while to get Jerry's things arranged in his bedroom so it would work for him. It also took some time to find good care providers to help him. Betty filled in as much as she could during those first few weeks.

As they had planned, Betty had a room at one end of the house and Jerry had a room at the other end. They had their computers, TV's, and their own projects to work on in their separate spaces. Then they shared meals in the kitchen. When nighttime came around, they would meet in the living room and watch TV. They had two dogs and Betty's cat who shared the various spaces in the house with them too.

That first summer was a rough one in the intense heat of the Central Valley. The house didn't have very good air conditioning and they would take naps and use fans to get through the hot afternoons. When they finally got a new swamp cooler, it helped a lot.

Jerry would go to the store and Betty sometimes added extra things to the list. Jerry wondered why they needed so many things when he was just going to the store for dinner. Back then, Betty had a sweet tooth. Also, Jerry could put away some serious bowls of ice cream.

One day, Jerry got the idea to get a large amount of canned fruit so he wouldn't have to go to the store so often. When he got home, he hit a stepping-stone that was in the way and over his chair went with him seat belted in it. The heavy cans of fruit had made his chair tip over on its back. He ended up on his back too.

Betty heard Jerry yelling for help, looked out the window, saw Jerry's legs in the air, and came running out to help him. A neighbor saw what happened too and ran over to help. Poor Jerry was on his back and his feet were in the air kicking. He wasn't hurt, luckily. This all happened right on top of my tunnels. The crash and all that kicking made the sides of my tunnels move. I checked and there wasn't any real damage. Jerry never again got that many cans of fruit.

Jerry wasn't easy to live with at times. Betty had gotten a wireless doorbell to keep next to his bed for Jerry to ring when he needed help. Well, one day, Jerry kept pushing it repeatedly for Betty to adjust his pillow. She had been trying to take a nap while Jerry was resting. And, of course, every time Jerry pushed the doorbell button next to his bed, the doorbell would ring in the kitchen and the dogs would bark thinking someone was at the door. The house had doorbells at the front door and kitchen doors too.

It was crazy there every time one of these doorbells went off. So, Betty never replaced the batteries, on the one near Jerry's bed, when they wore out, smart woman. She also got rid of the other doorbells too. To this day, she doesn't have a doorbell on her house.

Every night Jerry would come out of his room to have a snack. Well, once Betty was upset and yelled at Jerry. It scared him. Jerry tried to think of a way to slink back into his bedroom without Betty noticing him. But soon Betty calmed down and she fed Jerry his ice cream.

Betty and Jerry were up and down in their relationship. Jerry decided that it was time to have his own apartment. Jerry was ready to live on his own again. Jerry was always thankful for Betty taking him into her home and life.

Both Jerry and Betty were confused when Betty's mom said one day that it was a nice try. A nice try? They had done it for five years. Jerry and Betty thought it was a big accomplishment to have made it that long.

Betty is still his friend and care provider.

Section Four - Chapter 23 - BooBoo, Jerry's Dog

About two months after Jerry had moved in with Betty, she brought home a dog for him. Betty already had an Australian Shepherd named Sammie at this point and Boo was part Australian Shepherd too. This new puppy would give Sammie a buddy to keep her company and to play with in the yard. Sammie also took on the duty of being a mother to Boo because he was only three months old.

Jerry thought this new dog would be a lap dog that would quietly sit or lie by him. But was Jerry in for a surprise. This is what happened.

Betty was driving to the store and this puppy was in the street looking for someone to save him. When Betty opened the car door, that puppy didn't waste any time getting into the car. He knew a good thing when it came along. Someone had abandoned the puppy to live on the street.

The first time Jerry saw this new dog, it was very small and very scared. It just sat in a corner of the sofa trembling and shaking. Jerry went over to pet him. Jerry's hand and his heart went out to the small scared puppy.

Jerry named this dog Booboo or Boo for short. It was easy for Jerry to say. Also, Jerry thought Boo would understand his name when Jerry said it.

When Boo got older, the whole thing was different. It was obvious that Boo had decided at the very beginning to take over the house. So every body and everything in the house was his. He would go around sniffing and checking to see if everything and everybody was all right. Boo would lie in the middle of the hall where he could watch both Jerry and Betty who were in different rooms.

When Boo discovered that Jerry was able to give him dog cookies, it was on! Boo was very careful to take the cookie from Jerry's hand so as not to bite Jerry. Boo didn't want to hurt Jerry. Sometimes Jerry didn't know Betty had already given Boo cookies. But Boo would just sit in front of the cabinet where he knew the cookies were and look up at Jerry with his sad brown eyes. Boo had Jerry and everyone else that came into the house trained to get cookies from this cabinet. Of course, Sammie got a cookie too, every time Boo did this. She would be sitting right next to him waiting.

Boo really liked to play fetch with a ball. But, Jerry couldn't pick up the ball and throw it. So Boo would put the ball in Jerry's lap and Jerry would let the ball roll down his legs and into the yard. Boo would go get the ball and place it back into Jerry's lap so Jerry could roll it off again. That could go on for an hour. Boo never tired of playing this game with Jerry.

For over ten years, Boo and his buddy Sammie gave many laughs and much love and companionship to Betty and Jerry. Boo and Sammie kept things happening all the time. So, of course, no matter what it was, the dogs joined in. It was great fun living with the two dogs and Betty's cat, KC. Betty and Jerry still miss their critters.

Section Four - Chapter 24 - Mary Ann
Jerry's Friend and Care Provider

Jerry thought he would hire a care provider for part time. But it didn't work out that way. Mary Ann came along, became indispensable to Jerry, and has been a very important part of his life ever since.

Having Mary Ann working for Jerry gave Betty some freedom that she hadn't had before. Betty could go places and even travel occasionally with friends. When Betty was away, Mary Ann worked all hours of the day and night.

The three of them, Mary Ann, Betty, and Jerry started going on trips together. Betty and Jerry had traveled up and down California in the past, but it was getting difficult for Betty to do all the driving and all the care providing for Jerry too. She would get completely exhausted half way through a trip. Mary Ann and Betty took turns being care provider and this proved to be much easier on all of them. So, the three of them would go away on vacation almost every year.

They had trouble with most of the disabled bathrooms in the motels and restaurants they visited. I have to tell you about some of the bathrooms they had to deal with.

One time, Mary Ann had to have the motel remove the bathroom door to allow Jerry to get into the shower. The grab bar was so close to the wall that Jerry couldn't get his fingers around it to hold himself up while transferring. To top it off, Mary Ann and Betty still had to give Jerry sponge baths for the whole time they were there as the shower was unusable.

Because there was not enough room near the toilet, Betty could not help Mary Ann with Jerry when he needed to use the bathroom. Mary Ann had to hold him up and pull his pants down at the same time.

On another occasion, Betty had to call the motel office because when Jerry sat on the toilet the seat fell off on the floor. Jerry was left sitting on the rim of the toilet and holding on for dear life.

One time, Jerry wanted to go see something down the street. He didn't realize it was uphill all the way. Mary Ann pushed him there and back. That night Mary Ann wondered if this was in the contract she signed. If I know Jerry, he rewrote the contract. Jerry made up the rules as he went along, if he needed something from Mary Ann or anybody else.

Mary Ann did something that bothered Betty and Jerry when they went out to eat. Mary Ann cut up his food by chopping it with a knife or a fork and everybody in the restaurant was able to hear the knife and fork hitting the plate. Jerry looked the other way and acted as if he didn't know what was going on.

One night, Mary Ann came to feed Jerry some stew that Betty had made and it had a bay leaf in it. Mary Ann was going to take the bay leaf out of Jerry's mouth when she saw it, but he had already swallowed it. He started choking and coughing and did this for about 10 or 15 minutes. Mary Ann was about ready to call 911. But Jerry finally coughed and got the leaf out of his throat.

Mary Ann has a big heart. She would do anything for Jerry. But she was not able to remember things. Jerry had to tell her some things over and over.

When Jerry moved to his own apartment, Mary Ann didn't know how he would get by because he relied on Betty a lot. Mary Ann helped him move not one time but twice. She helped him move from Betty's house to the first apartment, which was too small and the bathroom wouldn't work for Jerry. Nothing would make it work either. No bars, no removing doors, nothing anyone could do to that bathroom would help. Jerry had to go to the bathroom using a commode in the shower. So, about two months later, Mary Ann had to move all of Jerry's stuff down the hall to a bigger apartment. She told Jerry that was it. She wouldn't move him anymore.

After Jerry moved into the second apartment, Mary Ann's husband came over to switch the large, heavy front doors. He took the door off the new apartment, moved it down the hall to the old apartment and then replaced the new door with the door from the old apartment. Jerry needed that door because he had bought and had installed a special expensive lock on it that enabled him to open the door using a remote control. The building management wouldn't let him switch the lock from one door to the other because they didn't want any holes drilled in the second door. The next morning the building management had to exchange the apartment numbers back and forth between the two doors. That was the easy part.

Later on, Mary Ann went to school with Jerry and helped him with his notebook, tape recorder, homework, and short story writing class assignments. School had always been a challenge for her.

One teacher saw the eagerness that Mary Ann expressed in learning to write short stories. The teacher began to work with her in the class. It was a very rewarding experience. The teacher would say something like, Jerry gets a "C" and Mary Ann gets an "A" today. In time, Mary Ann became comfortable in the classroom.

One time, no one else in the class knew an answer to a question the teacher had asked and Mary Ann held up her hand and said the correct answer. It was very hard for her to speak up in class. The teacher said, at least somebody listens to me. He said, next time you can leave Jerry home. Everybody in the class laughed. He smiled and went on with the class.

Jerry gave Mary Ann his old computer and in no time, Mary Ann was writing her own cookbook with recipes for meals for Jerry that wouldn't choke him. His speech problem was associated with a swallowing and choking problem.

These recipes looked and tasted good and gave Jerry more variety in his meals.

One night, before class, Jerry and Mary Ann were having coffee at the student café on campus. The teacher came in and sat down and Mary Ann showed him her cookbook. He actually looked through it for about ten minutes or so. After that, Mary Ann was on cloud nine. Jerry had to take a back seat to her cookbook.

Mary Ann was working for Jerry the last time I looked. That poor woman has to put up with that grumpy Jerry.

Section Four - Chapter 25 - Richard
Computer Guru and Jerry's Buddy

A short time after moving to central California, Jerry had problems with his computer. Betty sent Jerry's computer back east to the manufacturer for repairs. Those two or three weeks were unbearable for Betty because Jerry was lost for what to do without his computer. Jerry would follow Betty around the house asking unimportant questions such as what they were going to have for dinner. Even when Betty told him, he would, in a little while ask almost the same question again. Betty would suggest that he could go listen to books on tape. Jerry replied that he had already heard them all. Besides, he reminded Betty, he had moved there to be with her.

Needless to say, there were times when Betty wanted to do things to Jerry that weren't nice. From my viewpoint, as a gopher, I wouldn't have blamed her. I wanted to suggest some things such as putting a dirty washrag in his mouth. Jerry seemed to become ungrateful toward Betty and I was disappointed in him.

Shortly after, Jerry got his computer back and peace returned to the house. Jerry was in his room writing stories and Betty was far away in the other side of the house working on her watercolors. They both had wanted this life for a long time.

Then Jerry's computer was giving him trouble again. Neither Betty nor Jerry wanted to send it away leaving Jerry with nothing to do for two weeks. They both didn't think they would live through another period when Jerry didn't have his computer. And, as for myself, I couldn't stand to see them tear each other apart again. Besides, I had just begun to build a new room under the house. There were some neat things under that old house.

Just as it seemed to look like stressful times might be coming back, Jerry's social worker told him about a new computer lab at United Cerebral Palsy. At first, Jerry had his doubts about any program run by an agency. But, Betty had Jerry in the car before he could say anything.

I admire women who can take charge when a situation needs it. Like Betty, I couldn't be around Jerry again if he didn't have his computer working correctly. With this in mind, Betty took Jerry to United Cerebral Palsy and they met a lady named Kelly, who was the director of the adult day programs.

While the three were talking, Jerry noticed the man in the corner quietly doing something. Jerry couldn't really tell what the guy was doing but it spiked his curiosity. After a while, Kelly introduced the man in the corner and asked him to come over and meet everyone and this was the beginning of a long and beautiful relationship.

Jerry didn't know at the time but Richard, the man in the corner, was going to bring several great improvements into Jerry's life. It wouldn't only be better for Jerry but for Betty too. Jerry would be easier to live around when his computer worked the way he needed.

Jerry could use very few software programs. Even the programs made for people with disabilities couldn't do what he needed. Richard and Jerry would spend hours and hours looking on the internet for programs to help Jerry.

There were times when Richard would call Jerry's care provider to come take Jerry home and Richard and Jerry would work two more hours while the care provider waited. There were nights when the care provider wanted to kill both of them because Richard called before Jerry was ready to leave. It was hard to explain they had found something promising right after Richard called. The care provider only bought this excuse once. Richard and Jerry never knew about the plans the care provider had to hang the two of them.

Richard and Jerry together came up with many ways to improve Jerry's computer. Jerry wasn't able to read a newspaper so Richard came up with a computer program that turned text on the screen into digitized words that the computer read to Jerry and Jerry then was able to read three newspapers a day and two books a week.

At first, Jerry didn't know that Richard was a jokester. One day, Jerry had a fingernail that he needed to have someone trim for him. Richard told him just a minute and he would go get the lawnmower. Well, Jerry really believed everything Richard said. Jerry was always getting jokes played on him. One of Richard's jokes was always catching Jerry. Richard would say things in such a serious tone that Jerry would go for it almost every time. Once, I had to rush down a deep tunnel under United Cerebral Palsy to keep them from hearing me laugh.

As Jerry was always playing tricks on others, I was glad he had met his match. When Jerry was in the care facility, he would hide a spoon in his lap. Then when the orderly went and got another spoon Jerry would slip the first spoon back onto the table. The orderly became confused until he caught on to what Jerry was doing. Jerry had to do something for fun in that place. But I felt bad for the orderly.

Richard and Kelly had come up with an outreach program and invited teachers and the general public to come to the new computer lab they had set up. They opened the lab three hours each week free to anyone who came.

At this lab, people learned what the computer and the various software programs could offer those with disabilities. They also got to try various means of inputting information into the computer. Figuring out a workable alternative means of inputting information would often provide the breakthrough for a child to then be able to make use of what a computer could offer.

Richard would work one-on-one with a child who maybe could not use their fingers to type, to see if the child could hit a switch with the back of their hand or push a big button with their knee or use a head wand to hit keys on the computer keyboard. This takes a great deal of patience from all involved.

I set up a camera, with a long distance lens, in the wall of the computer room at United Cerebral Palsy. I thought I might as well pick up some pointers. After all, it was free to the public.

Jerry went each week to help with the computer lab project. Once, Jerry spoke a long time with a lady who had a three or four year old daughter. The lady was troubled about her daughter's future. Jerry merely listened to her story. Afterward, Jerry told a little about his past. He told how he had seen that things had improved for people with disabilities. The lady felt better and had more hope for her daughter's future.

One day, a little boy, who could not move his hands or legs, visited the lab. Several people worked with him, even Jerry, and they all gave up. Jerry went to help somebody else. Richard started working with the little boy. In an hour, Richard had the little boy typing his name. Some people that were there with the little boy went to another room and cried tears of happiness.

At one point, things had been slow for a few weeks at the lab. It was a period when people who might have needed help with computer issues just didn't come to the lab. There could have been a number of reasons for this. Teachers in special education didn't know that the computer lab was there. It was hard for people with disabilities to find a way to travel across town to the lab. Richard had people who would call to make appointments but then they wouldn't show up.

Then Richard had to do a report in order to request additional funding for the computer lab. There were others there that afternoon such as the speech pathologist who donated her time. Jerry had thought he would have a relaxing time sitting around talking with friends.   But, just as soon as his aid wheeled Jerry through the door, Richard came over and told him to get to work that he needed the report done and he needed Jerry's help to complete it.

Richard had already setup a computer and had Jerry's typing stick all ready for him in the low vision room where Jerry wouldn't be bothered. To tell the truth, Jerry was glad to write the report for Richard. Jerry was always looking for ways to repay people who had helped him. And Richard had helped him in so many ways.

Jerry had told everyone what a good writer he was. Now Jerry had to prove it. I rushed back to my tunnel room under the computer lab before someone could hear me laughing.

Each time Jerry came out of where he was working, with the hope of joining the group, Richard would send him back to work. Jerry could only come out to ask how to spell a certain word. At the end of the night, Jerry finished the report.

About every month or two, a college class of students would come to the computer lab. These were graduate students who were going into special education or studying to become speech pathologists. They would listen to Richard explain how some of the programs worked and how students at United Cerebral Palsy of Central California used these special computer programs.

Once, toward the end of his demonstration, Richard held up Jerry's plywood board with the letters of the alphabet on it. He explained to the students that in some instances that was all someone needed to communicate with those around them and not an expensive speech device. Jerry's letter board was very low tech but it worked for him. The fancy speech devices were beyond his ability to use because he had so little functional use of his hands.

Since Richard had used the letter board to end one demonstration, Jerry assumed Richard would end the next one the same way. But the letter board was way across the room. So Jerry, eager to help, picked up the plywood letter board, made his way through the crowd, and struggled to place the letter board on the table behind Richard. But, Richard, realizing he was running short on time, accidentally knocked the letter board on the floor and stepping on it asked if there were any questions. Jerry knew then that he, himself, would never make a very good prop man.

One time, the local TV station sent a reporter to do a story on the computer lab and all the computer programs that were out there for people with disabilities. The hope was to make the public more aware of the computer lab at United Cerebral Palsy of Central California. Richard wasn't very comfortable giving interviews so he brought the reporter to Jerry's apartment and Jerry showed the reporter how he used his computer that Richard designed and partly built. The reporter turned his demonstration into the interview. Jerry didn't know he had signed up to do public relations.

Richard and Jerry are still working together testing out computer software that may help Jerry and others like him.

Section Four - Chapter 26 - Going Back To College

About two years after moving to the Central Valley, Jerry decided to go back to school. He had been writing all along but he wanted to sharpen his skills. He figured going to City College would do it. Jerry was about fifty-eight and he was bored with life around home. The first class he signed up for was with Mr. Holmes. Jerry thought he was going to have it easy and he was right in a way. But, in other ways, going back to school was harder than he thought it would be.

Jerry met two other guys in the class who helped him in many ways. When the teacher passed around the first handout, Jerry wheeled across to one of his classmates asking for help to get the handout. It so happened that this guy was going to be a teacher for the disabled. But Jerry didn't know about that. The guy just helped Jerry with the handout. The other guy was a former Marine and sat in the back of the room. When the first guy didn't show up for class sometimes, the Marine would help Jerry. Sometimes the two guys would come early to read things to Jerry.

The teacher realized that Jerry needed to hear what the class was reading to themselves. But sometimes there wasn't enough time to read everything aloud because the class needed to move along. It was like a comedy of errors. One day the teacher joked aloud and asked the class if he was able to continue. Jerry told him go ahead. One guy said one minute and the teacher said half a minute.

During the lecture part of each class, the students would sit in a big circle around the room. When the teacher divided them into work groups, each group would move to a different corner of the classroom. The future special education teacher and the former Marine were in Jerry's work group.

When Jerry's group worked on a project, the guys would gather around Jerry and discuss what they needed to do. When one of the other groups started to come back to the circle, the guys would get all excited and ask them for another fifteen minutes. The teacher would jokingly say five. When they had finished the assignment, they would call to the other groups and say, "Okay, we're done."

After class, the Marine would help Jerry with his books and his tape recorder and put them in the bag hanging on Jerry's chair. Everybody else would just rush out. The Marine would get frustrated at their behavior, and ask himself, "How hard is it to help somebody?"

At the end of the class, some people got their stories printed in a book of student work that the college English Department published at the end of each year. There would be a get together and the people who had stories printed had a chance to read them aloud to the assembled people at the get together. Jerry had his story printed in the book and he asked the guy who was going to be a teacher to read his story.

Section Four - Chapter 27 - Jerry's Writing Teachers

When Jerry went back to school, he met two teachers there who believed in him and his writing ability. I thought Jerry merely wanted to see if he could still handle school. Instead, he got into more trouble than I thought was possible.

The first teacher was Mr. Holmes who taught the class described in the previous chapter. The first day of school, Jerry went with his care provider, Gloria, who was worried about getting him enrolled in the class. But Mr. Holmes said it would be no problem. When Jerry really started to enjoy school, this same care provider tried to make him late to class. That care provider just wanted Jerry to pay attention to her. Jerry was a good student in spite of that care provider.

Mr. Holmes didn't know what he was getting himself into either. After the first class, Jerry didn't have anybody to go with him to school. Jerry was moving his arms and hands to get the teacher's attention so he could tell him his ideas. Then Jerry was demonstrating, by flapping his arms up and down like a bird, that the characters were waiting for an airplane in Hemmingway's story, Hills like White Elephants. I stepped outside to laugh so I wouldn't disturb the class.

Jerry found that eventually people would get to know him as just another student. Then they would help him with reading his papers and books and even put them away for him at the end of class. One time, a guy was reading a handout to Jerry and made the whole class wait until he was done. Mr. Holmes, with a smile, asked Jerry if he could continue the class now and Jerry said, be my guest.

When Jerry was not enrolled in a class any longer, he would still stop by Mr. Holmes' office and Mr. Holmes would help Jerry with writing projects and answer any questions. Mr. Holmes always needed to use Jerry's letter board to understand what Jerry wanted to ask. Then Mr. Holmes would fold his arms and give Jerry a lecture on the subject right there on the sidewalk in front of his office.

One day Jerry asked Mr. Holmes about how to write an essay and got an easy to understand explanation from him. This helped to clarify some of the issues he had been having with his attempts to write essays. Mr. Holmes helped Jerry to enroll in an Independent Study class to learn how to get his work published. Jerry started writing essays on a regular basis and even got them published in the local newspaper.

After about two years, Mr. Holmes introduced Jerry to Mr. Fine, another teacher who taught short story writing. When Jerry signed up for Mr. Fine's short story writing class, Jerry started bringing Mary Ann, his care provider, to help him speak in class. This turned out to be a good idea and he continued taking her from then on.

Mr. Fine would make time for Jerry to speak but Jerry didn't know when that would be. It could be either at the beginning of the class, the middle, or towards the end of the class. When he did finally get to speak, and then was too long winded, Mr. Fine would say okay Jerry we are moving on now. Jerry would be about to say that he was not done yet but soon he knew that did not matter. The class moved on. Speech defect or not, Jerry sometimes wanted to talk too much.

One time, after both teachers had known Jerry for a while, Jerry would show up at one of their offices to ask a question. Mr. Fine would tell Jerry to go ask Mr. Holmes and Mr. Holmes would say go ask Mr. Fine. The next time Jerry went to visit Mr. Holmes, Mr. Holmes explained with a grin that he wasn't Jerry's teacher any more. Once, I became dizzy because Jerry was driving his power chair with me on the back between the two teachers' offices.

In time, Mr. Fine was the one who got Jerry back to writing short stories. Both of these teachers helped a great deal to improve Jerry's writing skills.

Section Four - Chapter 28 - You Won't Believe

Jerry had done some unusual things that most people, disabled or not, would not even think of doing. I will tell you some of the highlights.

George, who helped him move out of the "jail", as Jerry called the institution where he lived for ten years, would take him on vacations. One day, as they were walking thru the woods, Jerry asked George to put him in a tree. Before Jerry knew it, he was up in a tree on a limb. George took a picture of Jerry up in the tree. Jerry lost the photo so I am the only one that is able to say that it really happened.

Jerry had another friend named John and John put down boards on the sand at the beach so Jerry could roll over them in his wheelchair and cross the sand. Otherwise, the wheels on his wheelchair would just sink into the sand and he would get nowhere. If this wasn't enough, Jerry had another friend who Jerry had asked to help him walk by putting his feet in the sand. This was so Jerry could get the feeling of walking in sand. Before they knew it, Jerry's weight was too far foreword and they were running down the beach. They went quite a ways down the beach and it took a long time to walk back.

One time, Jerry's friend, John, took him to the movies. When they got there, they realized that there was no ramp for Jerry's chair to get up to the ticket booth. So Jerry told John to stand him up against the wall while John got Jerry's chair up on the sidewalk. Jerry didn't think about what would happen if he had fallen over. Sometimes Jerry didn't think about his actions. He just did what sounded good at the time.

There was the day Jerry went to the beach with a church group and one of the girls put two marshmallows in his mouth. He didn't know that his mouth was that big, but I did. You would think Jerry would be safe with a church group. But they all knew how he wanted to be a part of everything. Jerry looked around for a priest because he was choking on the marshmallows and thought he was going to die. About five years later, Jerry had an x-ray of his lungs. He had two masses or spots on his lungs and he told the technician that they were those marshmallows that he had choked on.

When Jerry was in the first care facility, George took him out for a walk to his car. Jerry thought it was just out in the back parking lot. But George had left it clear across town. George pushed Jerry, in his wheelchair, over the railroad tracks and down the walkway that ran next to the freeway to get to the car. People would pull over and ask if everything was okay. George would tell them that they were just going for a walk. Jerry did not know that George had done some dope just before he had arrived and they started their "walk." I was happy Jerry was able to make it home. It was hard sometimes to see why Jerry trusted George.

One afternoon, Jerry was coming home in his wheelchair and a car hit him. Jerry was able to move out of the way enough, just in time, so he didn't get hurt. A neighbor, who knew Jerry, came out of his house. He helped Jerry up over the curb, got his letter board, and asked Jerry if he was all right. The policeman, who came to the scene, just wanted Jerry's identification. The policeman was more worried about the car than Jerry. Unfortunately, a city employee driving a city owned vehicle had hit him. Another policeman came and took pictures of Jerry's chair. Jerry thought somebody would help him pay for repairs to his power wheelchair. But the police report said that it was Jerry's fault and the city denied any responsibility. Jerry wanted so badly to go hit a police car but he didn't want to chance being arrested.

A few years later, another car hit Jerry, when he went to the Echo Café for coffee one evening. Everybody in the café knew Jerry and they all came outside and wanted to tear the car apart. Jerry could have made a problem out of it but it would not be good for the image of the disabled. Jerry was on the Board of Directors at United Cerebral Palsy and he figured that this was not what they meant about getting more publicity for the organization and raising awareness in the community about its programs.

Most evenings, Jerry would go to the Echo Café for coffee and to listen to local musicians. Those people didn't look at Jerry as being a disabled guy. One day, they asked Jerry to play the banjo. Jerry said that he was just a writer and that it would be hard to get the banjo on his lap. But, he actually did it and strummed the strings and the guy told him to come back anytime. I was happy that Jerry didn't try to play the whole song on the banjo. It would have hurt my ears.

Epilogue

Epilogue
By Frank, "The Gopher"

Looking back at all the things that Jerry did I am amazed at how he made it through some of them. While keeping up with Jerry over these years, I learned that all the people in his life were instrumental in helping him to accomplish the things he did. And I feel privileged to have had the opportunity to be there and witness events as they unfolded.

I just heard Jerry leaving his apartment. I don't want to miss what Jerry will be doing next. I am shutting down my computer and continuing my commitment to *Keeping Up With Jerry*.